Questions & Answers

O LEVEL
HUMAN BIOLOGY

D. Reese
B.Sc.(Hons), Cert.Ed.

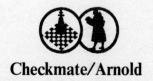

Checkmate/Arnold

First published in Great Britain 1986 by
Checkmate Publications,
4 Ainsdale Close, Bromborough, Wirral L63 0EU.

This edition published in association with
Edward Arnold (Publishers) Ltd.,
41 Bedford Square, London WC1B 3DQ

Edward Arnold (Australia) Pty Ltd.,
80 Waverley Road, Caulfield East,
Victoria 3145, Australia

Edward Arnold, 3 East Read Street,
Baltimore, Maryland 21202, USA.

ISBN 0 946973 26 1

Printed and bound by Richard Clay (The Chaucer Press),
Bungay, Suffolk

TABLE OF CONTENTS

PAGE NUMBER

INTRODUCTION

This book is intended to be a revision aid. It is designed to be used to supplement a text book or notes obtained from a course in human biology.

The **questions** given have been carefully selected to provide a full coverage of the main topic areas. They have been based closely upon recent O level questions set by a number of examination boards.

The **answers** should not be interpreted as providing a perfect model, which if copied would produce a guaranteed grade "A" in an examination. They are intended to give you a guide on how to set about answering many of the most common examination questions.

To obtain the best use of the material in this book you should **first** familiarise yourself with a topic, e.g. respiration. **Then** choose a question from the book. After you have attempted the question **compare** your answer with the one given in the back of the book.

Finally, at the end of each topic a list of **key words** are given. When you have completed your revision you should be familiar with the meaning of each word in the list.

The following are some points that should be remembered when attempting different types of questions:

General points
1. Ensure that you have **read** the question carefully before beginning your answer.
2. Attempt to keep your answers **concise,** you do not gain credit for the length of your answer, simply for the facts that it contains.
3. The **number of marks** allocated to a question are a useful indication of the number of separate points required in your answer. Use them to judge the detail needed in the answer.
4. Whenever possible give **examples** to help explain your answer.
5. When answering an "essay" type question (e.g. describe the digestion of a piece of lean meat. Q16) always begin by writing a brief **plan** of the topics you intend to cover.
6. At the end of your answer, always **total** up the marks awarded for each portion of the question. **Check** that your marks correspond with the total marks allocated for the whole question.

7. Always attempt each part of a question.
8. Indicate **clearly** which parts of a question you are attempting (e.g. Q13a(ii)).

When using diagrams
1. Always use a sharpened pencil (**never** a pen).
2. Do not colour diagrams in.
3. Use shading **selectively,** only where it helps to **clarify** your diagram.
4. Draw **large, clear** diagrams which are **fully labelled.**
5. **Print** your labels and ensure that the lines do not cross over each other.
6. Put a **title** below your diagram.
7. If asked to draw a diagram, the number of marks given, give an **indication** of the number of labels required.

When plotting graphs
1. Always **label** the **axes** clearly (e.g. time, weight etc.)
2. Always **state** the **units** used (e.g. seconds, kilogrammes etc.)
3. Always **state** the **title** of the graph (e.g. changes in body temperature with time).
4. Mark your points **accurately** using a sharpened pencil.

When attempting a calculation
1. Set your work out neatly and show the **stages** in your calculation clearly.
2. If you make an error put a single line through the mistake. Do not scribble it out so that the examiner is unable to see what you have done.
3. Use the **correct units** throughout your calculation.

When describing experiments
1. Describe the experiment under the following headings:— **Aim (or title), Apparatus, Method, Results, Conclusion.**

QUESTION 1   p32

(a) Draw a large labelled diagram of a typical animal cell as seen with a light microscope.   *(3 marks)*

(b) In what ways do each of the following types of cell differ from the cell you have drawn. How is the structure of each related to its function?

   i)   Sperm cell.   *(3 marks)*

   ii) Red blood cell (Erythrocyte).   *(3 marks)*

   iii) Sensory neurone.   *(3 marks)*

(c) Explain the function of Deoxyribonucleic acid, Ribonucleic acid, Ribosomes and Mitochondria in the formation of protein.   *(6 marks)*

(d) State precisely in the body where each of the following types of cells could be found:

   i)   One which stores glycogen.

   ii) One which produces Hydrochloric acid.

   iii) One that secretes a calcium compound around itself.

   iv) One that contains a pigment called visual purple (Rhodopsin).   *(2 marks)*

(Total 20 marks)

QUESTION 2   p34

(a) i) What is meant by the term an organelle? Give two examples of organelles found in all animal cells.
                                                           (3 marks)

   ii) What is meant by the term a tissue.   *(1 mark)*

(b) Give examples of the position in the body of the following tissues along with a description of their structure when viewed under a light microscope.

   i)   Ciliated epithelium.   *(4 marks)*

   ii) Compact bone.   *(6 marks)*

4

iii) Involuntary (smooth, unstriped) muscle. *(3 marks)*

(c) What are chromosomes? Where in the cell are they found. How many chromosomes are found in a liver cell and an erythrocyte (a red blood cell)? *(4 marks)*

(Total 20 marks)

QUESTION 3

p37p37

(a) One of the main functions of the skin is protection. Explain how the skin can protect the body against each of the following:

i) Ultra-violet light. *(3 marks)*

ii) Water loss. *(2 marks)*

iii) Entry of bacteria. *(2 marks)*

iv) Development of rickets. *(3 marks)*

(b) What is considered to be normal body temperature. *(1 mark)*

(c) Where is the body's temperature control centre. *(1 mark)*

(d) On a hot summer's day the skin produces a lot of sweat. Explain the value and consequences of this action. *(4 marks)*

(e) Explain why it is advisable to wear light coloured, loose fitting clothes in the summer. *(4 marks)*

(Total 20 marks)

QUESTION 4

The graph below shows the temperature of a person before, during and following a cold bath. The temperature was recorded in the mouth.

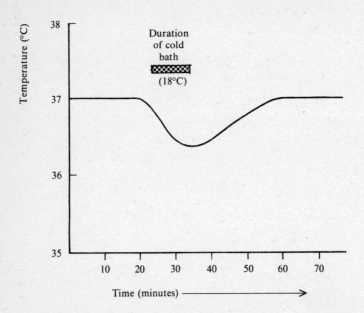

(a) i) When the person entered the cold bath the temperature of the external environment is much lower than that of the body. State **two** pathways by which the central nervous system is informed of the change. *(4 marks)*

   ii) Describe **two** changes in the body caused by entering the cold bath which help the temperature to return to normal. *(2 marks)*

(b) Strenuous exercise may cause light coloured skin to take on a much deeper pink appearance.

   i) Describe the changes which occur in the skin to cause this appearance. *(2 marks)*

   ii) What is the functional significance of this change. *(2 marks)*

(c) Body temperature is regulated at 36.9°C, and varies little from this point. This temperature is maintained by a balance between heat gained and heat lost by the body.

    i) List two ways in which the body gains heat and two ways in which heat can be lost. *(4 marks)*

(d) Explain each of the following:

    i) Although subject to constant friction the skin seldom wears away. *(4 marks)*

    ii) The skin can be thought of as an excretory organ. *(2 marks)*

(Total 20 marks)

QUESTION 5 p39

(a) i) Draw a **large,** clearly labelled diagram of a **named** hinge joint in a limb. *(9 marks)*

    ii) An antagonistic pair of muscles is needed for movement at this joint. Explain concisely the meaning of this statement. *(5 marks)*

(b) When lifting a heavy object from the ground you are advised to bend the knees keeping your back straight, and not to bend the back. Explain why this is good advice. *(4 marks)*

(c) State two functions of the skeleton (other than for muscle attachment. *(2 marks)*

(Total 20 marks)

QUESTION 6 p40

(a) Describe one example of how the bones in the limbs can act as a lever. *(4 marks)*

(b) State the differences in the properties of ligaments and tendons and explain the need for these differences. *(4 marks)*

(c) The diagram below shows a superior (anterior) view of a lumbar vertebra.

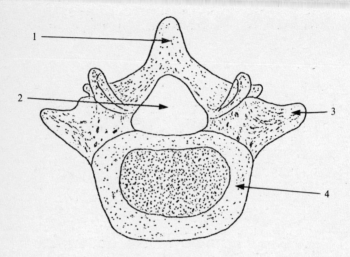

i) Name the numbered parts. *(4 marks)*

ii) What is the functional importance of part 2?
(1 mark)

(d) Name two types of joint other than a synovial joint. For each joint state one situation where it is found in the body. *(4 marks)*

(e) Wearing high heeled shoes causes the body weight to be pushed forward onto the balls of the feet. State 3 possible harmful effects that could be produced by excessive use of this type of footwear. *(3 marks)*

(Total 20 marks)

QUESTION 7 p42

(a) Describe the stages in the formation of urine.
(10 marks)

(b) The graph shows the results of some early experiments performed to investigate the functions of the liver and the kidneys.

Concentration of urea in blood
(mg per dm³)

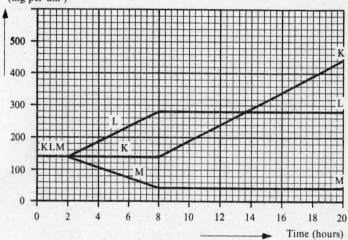

Graph **K** — kidneys removed after 8 hours.

Graph **L** — kidneys removed after 2 hours and the liver removed after 8 hours.

Graph **M** — liver removed after 2 hours and the kidneys removed after 8 hours.

i) Suggest what the concentration of the urea in the blood would be at 20 hours if no organs had been removed. *(1 mark)*

ii) State the concentration of urea in the blood at 20 hours for each of the graphs **L** and **M**. *(2 marks)*

iii) Using your knowledge of the functions of the liver and the kidney explain the differences between graphs **L** and **M**. *(7 marks)*

(Total 20 marks)

QUESTION 8 p44

(a) The diagram below shows a cross section of part of the coiled tubule of a nephron with a capillary attached.

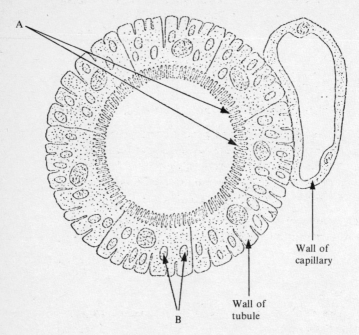

Wall of capillary

Wall of tubule

B

i) Of what advantage are the structures labelled A to the functioning of the tubule? *(1 mark)*

ii) Both the tubule and capillary are only one cell thick. What is the advantage of this to the functioning of the tubule? *(1 mark)*

iii) Identify structures B and briefly explain their importance to the functioning of the tubule.

(2 marks)

(b) The volume of the filtrate produced by the kidneys from the blood is about 120 cm³ per minute. Urine leaves the kidneys at the rate of about 1 cm³ per minute.

i) Briefly describe how the volume of this filtrate is reduced in the formation of urine. *(3 marks)*

ii) Name two substances which are normally present in the filtrate but not in the urine. *(2 marks)*

iii) Name one component of the blood plasma which is not present in either filtrate or urine. Briefly explain the reason for its absence from the filtrate.
(3 marks)

(c) It may be noticed that a greater volume of urine is produced in cold weather than in hot weather, although the diet remains constant.

i) Explain the reason for this phenomenon. *(3 marks)*

ii) Name the principal nitrogenous compound present in urine. Why does urine which is produced in cold weather have a lower concentration of this substance compared with urine produced in hot weather, providing the diet is unchanged? *(2 marks)*

(d) Micturition in babies is a simple reflex action. Explain what is meant by this statement. *(3 marks)*

(Total 20 marks)

QUESTION 9   p45

(a) i) Describe the functioning of the mechanism by which air is drawn into the lungs. *(5 marks)*

(b) i) Explain what is meant by the term tissue respiration.
(2 marks)

ii) Briefly state the role and relationships to each other of adenosine triphosphate (ATP) and adenosine diphosphate (ADP) in tissue respiration. *(4 marks)*

(c) The table below shows some results obtained in an experiment when a person at rest breathed air containing different amounts of carbon dioxide.

% carbon dioxide in inspired air	0.04	1.50	3.10	6.00
Tidal volume (cm³)	520	720	1190	2100
Breathing rate (breaths per minute)	14	15	16	28

i) What is the usual percentage of carbon dioxide in normal air. *(1 mark)*

ii) What is the effect on breathing of inspiring increased concentrations of carbon dioxide? *(2 marks)*

iii) What is the volume of air breathed in per minute when breathing 0.04% carbon dioxide and when breathing 6.00% carbon dioxide? *(2 marks)*

iv) Air breathed in contains about 20% oxygen. Of the oxygen taken into the lungs about 20% is used by the body. Calculate the amount of oxygen being used by the body each minute when breathing 0.04% carbon dioxide. Show your working. *(3 marks)*

(d) What part of the brain controls the breathing rate and tidal volume? *(1 mark)*

(Total 20 marks)

QUESTION 10   p47

The graph below shows different lung volumes for a person based on a number of spirometer recordings.

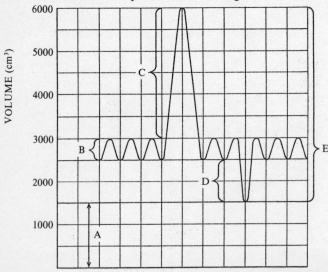

(a) Using information given on the graph, state the value of each of the following, along with the letter which represents it:

i) Inspiratory reserve volume.

ii) Vital capacity.

iii) Residual volume. *(6 marks)*

(b) i) What is meant by the term "tidal volume"?
(2 marks)

ii) Of the air taken in with each breath around 150 cm³ does not reach the gaseous exchange surfaces of the lungs. Briefly suggest a reason for this. *(3 marks)*

(c) Describe an experiment which may be used to compare the amount of carbon dioxide in inspired and expired air. Your account should include a description (or drawing) of the apparatus, reagents used, and the method of using this apparatus. Briefly indicate the results which you would expect. *(6 marks)*

(d) State three ways in which the alveoli are adapted to carry out gas exchange. *(3 marks)*

(Total 20 marks)

QUESTION 11

(a) The diagram shows an apparatus which may be used to demonstrate some of the features of the mechanism of breathing.

p48

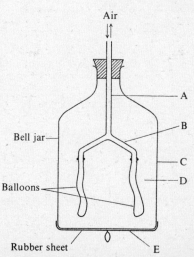

i) When the rubber sheet is pulled down, a small amount of air enters the balloons, causing them to inflate slightly. Explain the reason for this. *(4 marks)*

ii) Name those structures of the thorax which are represented in the apparatus by the letters A to E.
(5 marks)

iii) Briefly describe **five** ways in which the apparatus is a poor representation of the structure of the thorax.
(5 marks)

(b) What is meant by the term "anaerobic respiration"? Where in the body does it occur and under what conditions? *(3 marks)*

(c) After a subject has performed strenuous exercise, it is said that he must then repay his "oxygen debt". Briefly explain this statement. *(3 marks)*

(Total 20 marks)

QUESTION 12 p49

(a) Describe the method of functioning of an alveolus.
(8 marks)

(b) State two differences in the composition of blood flowing in the pulmonary artery and the pulmonary vein.
(2 marks)

(c) i) State two effects which vigorous exercise will have on breathing. *(2 marks)*

ii) Athletic training, involving regular strenuous exercise over a long period can affect breathing. State the changes which may occur. *(3 marks)*

iii) **Briefly** outline the main harmful effects associated with cigarette smoking. *(5 marks)*

(Total 20 marks)

14

(a) On investigating the energy loss by a human the following results were recorded:

Heat loss from body =	9800 kilojoules in 24 hours
Energy loss in urine =	380 kilojoules in 24 hours

Energy release in the same 24-hour period by the oxidation of ingested food:

From oxidation of carbohydrates =	3540 kilojoules
From oxidation of fats =	2390 kilojoules
From oxidation of proteins =	1880 kilojoules

    i) By how much does the energy utilised exceed the energy available from the food ingested? *(2 marks)*

    ii) The energy deficit is made available from food reserves. Name two food reserve materials and for each state one organ in which it is stored in humans. *(4 marks)*

(b) Give a brief explanation of the following statements:

    i) Fluoride is added to the public water supply.

                                                 (3 marks)

    ii) The amount of vitamin D needed in the diet of different individuals varies greatly. *(3 marks)*

    iii) Food such as citrus fruits, tomatoes or green salads are included in most diets. *(2 marks)*

    iv) Roughage (dietary fibre) has no energy or nutritional value but is still an essential component of the diet. *(3 marks)*

(c) What is meant by the term "a balanced diet".

                                                     (3 marks)

(Total 20 marks)

QUESTION 14

p53

Hydrogen peroxide can be decomposed by catalysts into water and oxygen. In an experiment investigating this, samples of the following fresh and previously boiled materials were added to samples of hydrogen peroxide. Any gas evolved was tested with a glowing splint.

Test-tube	Contents	Test on gas evolved
1	Hydrogen peroxide	No oxygen evolved
2	Hydrogen peroxide + fresh manganese dioxide	Oxygen evolved
3	Hydrogen peroxide + boiled manganese dioxide	Oxygen evolved
4	Hydrogen peroxide + fresh liver	Oxygen evolved
5	Hydrogen peroxide + boiled liver	No oxygen evolved
6	Hydrogen peroxide + fresh blood	Oxygen evolved
7	Hydrogen peroxide + boiled blood	No oxygen evolved

(a) i) For what reason is tube **1** set up? *(2 marks)*

ii) Explain precisely what is happening in tube **2** and what is causing this. *(2 marks)*

iii) Explain the results which occur in tubes **4** and **6**. *(2 marks)*

iv) Explain the results obtained in tubes **5** and **7**. *(4 marks)*

v) Explain the result obtained in tube **2**.

vi) State **two** factors which should be kept constant in all seven tubes. *(2 marks)*

(b) i) Draw a labelled diagram of a villus. *(4 marks)*

ii) Use your diagram to describe the absorption of glucose, fatty acids and glycerol from the small intestine. *(3 marks)*

(Total 20 marks)

QUESTION 15 p55

(a) For each of the following blood vessels state where it originates and where it terminates.

   i) Hepatic artery.

   ii) Hepatic vein.
   iii) Hepatic portal vein.   *(6 marks)*

(b) List three differences in the composition of blood flowing in the hepatic artery and the hepatic vein.
(3 marks)

(c) List three differences between the composition of blood in the hepatic portal vein and the hepatic vein shortly after a meal.   *(3 marks)*

(d) Why is blood vessel iii) different to most of the other blood vessels in the body?   *(1 mark)*

(e) i) Which two organs produce secretions which are passed into the duodenum?   *(2 marks)*

   ii) Describe how these secretions are involved in the digestion of fats.   *(5 marks)*

(Total 20 marks)

QUESTION 16 p56

(a) Describe the stages in the digestion of a piece of lean meat (you may assume that the meat contains no fat).
(12 marks)

(b) What is peristalsis and how is the structure of the alimentary canal adapted for this process?   *(8 marks)*

(Total 20 marks)

QUESTION 17 p58

(a) Distinguish between the following terms:

   i) A lymphocyte and a granulocyte (phagocyte or polymorphonucleocyte).   *(6 marks)*

ii) Antibodies and antigens. *(6 marks)*

iii) Serum and a vaccine. *(6 marks)*

(b) State two functions of the lymphatic system. *(2 marks)*

(Total 20 marks)

QUESTION 18   p60

(a) i) Explain how agglutinogens (antigens) and agglutinins (antibodies) are related to each other to produce the blood groups A, B, AB and O. *(7 marks)*

ii) If you were provided with a sample of blood, briefly describe how you would determine its blood group using serum from group A blood and from group B blood. *(5 marks)*

(b) In the form of a table state **three** differences in the structure of arteries and veins. *(3 marks)*

(c) In the form of a list describe the path followed by an erythrocyte (red blood cell) as it leaves the liver until it enters a kidney. (Include the chambers of the heart through which it passes). *(5 marks)*

(Total 20 marks)

QUESTION 19   p62

(a) The diagram shows a ventral external view of the heart.

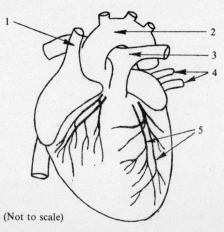

(Not to scale)

i) Name the blood vessels labelled **1, 2, 3** and **4,** and for each state whether the blood flowing through it is oxygenated or deoxygenated. *(4 marks)*

ii) Identify the blood vessels labelled **5.** Explain briefly the role they play in the functioning of the heart. *(2 marks)*

iii) Describe the sequence of events occurring in the heart which maintains the movement of blood from its entry into the right atrium (auricle) to its exit from the right ventricle. *(7 marks)*

(b) List the main stages in the clotting of blood. *(7 marks)*

(Total 20 marks)

QUESTION 20   p63

(a) Briefly describe the main functions of blood. *(8 marks)*

(b) Explain each of the following:

i) The function of the valves found in the circulatory system. *(6 marks)*

ii) How blood flow is maintained through veins. *(4 marks)*

iii) The sound of the heart beat is often described as being "Lubb dupp". *(2 marks)*

(Total 20 marks)

QUESTION 21   p65

(a) i) Give two characteristics of a reflex action. *(2 marks)*

ii) If a hot object is accidentally touched the hand is rapidly withdrawn. Describe in detail the mechanism of this reflex action beginning with the stimulation by the hot object. *(9 marks)*

iii) If a person had consumed a quantity of alcohol before touching the hot object, how would this have affected their response? *(2 marks)*

(b)   The diagram is a sectional view of the brain.

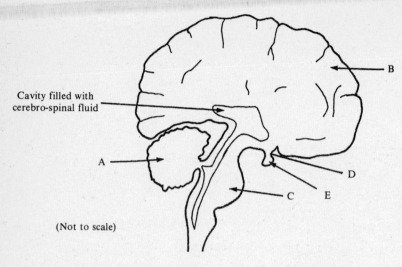

Cavity filled with
cerebro-spinal fluid

B

A

C   E

D

(Not to scale)

i)   Briefly describe the main functions of the parts
labelled **A**, **B**, **C** and **D**.   *(4 marks)*

ii)   Name the part labelled **E**.   *(1 mark)*

iii) The nervous system contains grey matter and white
matter. Briefly explain the reason for the difference
in appearance of these two.   *(2 marks)*

(Total 20 marks)

QUESTION 22   p67

(a)   The diagram represents a simplified vertical section
through the eye:

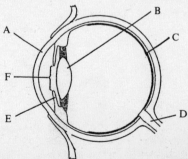

A

B

C

F

E

D

(Not to scale)

i) Name the parts labelled **A, B, C, D, E** and **F**.
(3 marks)

ii) State the function of each of the parts labelled **A, B, C** and **D**.
(4 marks)

iii) Describe the changes which occur in **E** and **F** when a person moves from bright sunlight into a heavily shaded area.
(3 marks)

iv) What is the value of the action described in iii) to the eye?
(1 mark)

(b) A person looking into the distance focuses his eye on a near object, for example this page. Describe the changes which have occurred in the eye so that the near object may be seen clearly. (Ignore movements of the eyeball and adjustments for changes in light intensity).
(6 marks)

(c) Briefly explain the advantage to humans of having overlapping fields of view.
(3 marks)

(Total 20 marks)

QUESTION 23
p68

(a) i) Draw a simple, fully labelled diagram to show image formation in the eye of a person with hypermetropia (long sight).
(4 marks)

ii) Draw a second diagram to show how this condition can be corrected with a suitable lens.
(2 marks)

(b) The diagram shows the chemical changes which occur in a rod cell in the retina.

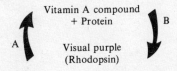

State which change — **A** or **B**

i) occurs when light passes into the cell

ii) produces a nerve impulse

iii) requires a supply of adenosine triphosphate (ATP).
(3 marks)

(c) i) In good light intensity both shape and colour can be seen, but in low light intensity whilst form may still be seen colour is difficult to distinguish. Account for this. *(6 marks)*

ii) Explain why a faint object such as a dim star, may be seen more clearly if it is not looked at directly.
(5 marks)

(Total 20 marks)

QUESTION 24

p69

(a) What are the ossicles and what is their function?
(4 marks)

(b) Describe the internal structure of the cochlea and explain how vibrations of the oval window lead to nerve impulses being transmitted along the auditory nerve. *(10 marks)*

(c) Briefly explain why a heavy cold can lead to partial deafness. *(3 marks)*

(d) Where in the body can an ampulla be found and how is it similar to the organ of corti found in the cochlea?
(3 marks)

(Total 20 marks)

QUESTION 25

p72

(a) i) Draw a simple, labelled diagram showing the position in the body of the main endocrine glands.
(6 marks)

ii) For each gland state **one** hormone that it produces. *(3 marks)*

iii) State **three** general properties of all hormones.
(3 marks)

(b) In the medical condition Diabetes, the patient suffers from a deficiency of a hormone which helps to control the blood glucose concentration.

   i) Name the hormone which is deficient and the endocrine gland that would normally produce it. *(2 marks)*

   ii) Briefly explain the function of this hormone. *(3 marks)*

(c) Which hormone when released into the bloodstream produces "the Fight or Flight Response". Give **two** effects which it produces in the body. *(3 marks)*

(Total 20 marks)

QUESTION 26   p73

The diagram represents a section through the male reproductive system.

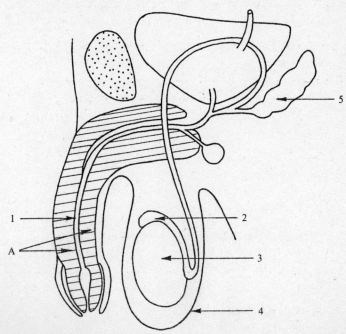

(a) Identify and state the function of each of the parts labelled **1, 2, 3, 4** and **5**. *(11 marks)*

(b) What is the nature of the tissue labelled **A**. Give a brief account of the importance and function of this tissue. *(4 marks)*

(c) In the early stages of development of a foetus, the testes are formed inside the abdomen. They then gradually descend to their normal position. In some cases this process is not complete at the time of birth. If this situation was not corrected explain the effects this would produce on the man's fertility. *(3 marks)*

(d) Briefly explain the difference between the terms semen and sperm. *(2 marks)*

(Total 20 marks)

QUESTION 27 p74
(a) Draw a labelled diagram to represent the female reproductive system. *(6 marks)*

(b) On your diagram label the following points with the appropriate letter:

i) Where sperm are deposited — Letter A

ii) Where fertilisation normally occurs — Letter B

iii) Where follicle stimulating hormone has its action — Letter C *(3 marks)*

(c) The menstrual cycle is controlled by the hormones oestrogen and progesterone. Briefly describe the differences between these two hormones in relation to where and at what stage during the cycle they are formed and released, along with their effects on the lining of the uterus. *(8 marks)*

(d)   The diagram below represents a simple view of the stages which may lead to pregnancy:

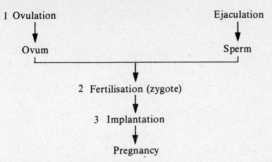

Describe three different methods of contraception, which act by preventing steps 1, 2 or 3.   *(3 marks)*

(Total 20 marks)

QUESTION 28   p76

(a)   Briefly state the path followed by a sperm from the time it enters the female's body until fertilisation occurs.
                                                        (3 marks)

(b)   What is meant by the following terms?

   i)   Ovulation

   ii)   Fertilisation

   iii) Implantation.   *(6 marks)*

(c)   i)   The placenta is an organ of gas exchange, excretion and nutrition. State **three** differences, one relating to each of these functions, between the composition of blood flowing in the umbilical artery and the umbilical vein.   *(3 marks)*

   ii)   The blood of the mother and the foetus do not mix normally. State **three** reasons why this is important to the foetus.   *(3 marks)*

   iii) In what ways is the circulation of the foetus different from that of an adult? What changes take place shortly after birth?   *(5 marks)*

(Total 20 marks)

25

QUESTION 29

(a) The diagram shows a vertical section of a mammary gland.

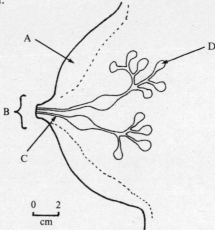

0   2
cm

   i)   Name the parts labelled **A, B, C** and **D**.   *(4 marks)*

   ii) What is colostrum?

   iii) Give **three** advantages to the child of being breast fed.   *(3 marks)*

   iv) Human milk provides almost all nutrients needed for a balanced diet. State the one nutrient which it lacks and why a healthy new born baby does not show any symptoms of a deficiency in this substance.

                                                        (2 marks)

(b) Oxytocin and prolactin are associated with birth and lactation. State where they are produced and their functions.   *(4 marks)*

(c) Briefly explain the following:

   i)   amniocentesis.   *(2 marks)*

   ii) the function of amniotic fluid.   *(3 marks)*

   iii) Breast fed babies usually lose weight for the first few days after birth.   *(2 marks)*

                                        (Total 20 marks)

QUESTION 30   p79

The graph shows the average heights for males and females up to the age of twenty.

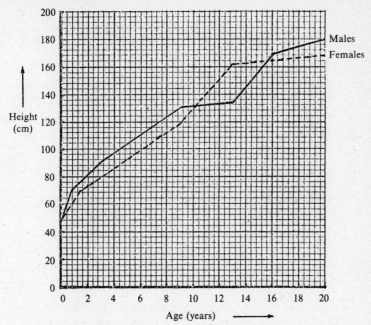

(a) Use the graph above to answer the following:—

    i)   During which four years do males show their slowest rate of growth?   *(1 mark)*

    ii) What are the average heights of a fully grown male and female?   *(2 marks)*

    iii) What is the average height of a 12-year old male?   *(1 mark)*

    iv) At what ages are males and females the same average height?   *(2 marks)*

(b) Between the ages of 10-13 years in girls and 13-16 years in boys rapid changes occur in the body.

    i)   What is this stage in development known as?   *(1 mark)*

ii) During this stage the secondary sexual characteristics develop. Briefly describe the main changes that occur in males and the hormone which is responsible for controlling them. *(8 marks)*

(c) Briefly describe the major factors which determine the rate of growth in height and the final height achieved. *(5 marks)*

(Total 20 marks)

QUESTION 31   p80

(a) Explain briefly the meaning of the following terms:

   i) Homologous chromosomes. *(2 marks)*

   ii) Chromatid and centromere. *(4 marks)*

   iii) Chiasmata. *(2 marks)*

(b) Mitosis and meiosis are both types of cell division.

   i) Briefly state the differences between a cell produced by mitosis and one produced by meiosis. *(4 marks)*

   ii) State two organs in the body, one where mitosis and one where meiosis occurs. *(2 marks)*

(c) Birth rate statistics show that approximately the same number of males and females are born each year. Using your knowledge of human biology explain why this is so. *(6 marks)*

(Total 20 marks)

QUESTION 32   p82

(a) The inheritance of the Rhesus blood factor is determined by a pair of alleles. Inheritance of the dominant allele results in the formation of the Rhesus antigen on the surface of red blood cells, causing Rhesus positive blood.

   i) What are the possible phenotypes and genotypes that can occur in the population? *(5 marks)*

ii) By means of a fully labelled diagram show how it is possible for a father and mother who are both Rhesus positive to have a child who is Rhesus negative.

(5 marks)

What is the probability of their child being Rhesus negative? *(1 mark)*

iii) By means of a fully labelled diagram show how a Rhesus negative mother could have a baby who is Rhesus positive. *(4 marks)*

iv) If this mother should have a second Rhesus positive baby it may have a type of anaemia caused by the Rhesus factor. Concisely explain how this may be caused. *(5 marks)*

(Total 20 marks)

QUESTION 33   p84

(a) The inheritance of the A, B, O blood groups are controlled by 3 alleles. The allele for group O blood is recessive to the alleles for group A and B. The alleles for A and B blood groups are said to show incomplete dominance (co-dominance)?

  i) What is meant by the term "incomplete dominance" (co-dominance)? *(3 marks)*

  ii) A woman of group A blood gives birth to a child of group O blood. The mother claims that a man of group B blood is the father. Is this possible? Fully explain your answer. *(6 marks)*

(b) i) Some conditions such as haemophilia are said to be "sex linked". What is meant by this term? *(2 marks)*

  ii) The allele for the condition haemophilia, h, is recessive to that for normal blood clotting, H. Describe the possible genotypes for males and females who do not suffer from haemophilia. *(3 marks)*

iii) What is meant by the term "a carrier female"? Describe the possible offspring produced if a carrier female marries a male with normal blood clotting.

(6 marks)

(Total 20 marks)

QUESTION 34   p87

(a) Explain the difference between refuse and sewage.

(2 marks)

(b) Briefly explain the biological reasons for burying refuse. *(3 marks)*

(c) The refuse buried in a tip will reduce in volume by up to 60% after a period of time.

  i) Explain what is happening to this refuse. *(2 marks)*

  ii) Explain what is likely to make up the remaining 40%. *(2 marks)*

(d) Describe and explain the main stages in the treatment of sewage. *(11 marks)*

(Total 20 marks)

QUESTION 35   p89

(a) What is meant by the term "potable water"? *(2 marks)*

(b) Explain concisely the effect of the following processes used in the treatment of river water to make it fit for human consumption.

  i) Sedimentation *(3 marks)*

  ii) Sand filtration. *(3 marks)*

  iii) Chlorination (sterilisation). *(2 marks)*

(c) Much of the water drunk in large towns has been drunk or used before. It is treated at sewage works before being passed back into lakes and rivers.

i) Give two diseases that could be transmitted through passing untreated sewage into a river. *(2 marks)*

ii) What would be the effect on animal life in a river if untreated sewage was discharged in large quantities. *(3 marks)*

(d) Explain the biological reason for each of the following statements.

i) Food scraps should be wrapped before being placed in a dustbin. *(2 marks)*

ii) A frozen chicken should be thoroughly thawed before cooking. *(4 marks)*

(Total 20 marks)

QUESTION 36   p90

(a) Describe how each of the following methods help to preserve the storage life of food:

i) Addition of salt. *(3 marks)*

ii) Canning. *(3 marks)*

iii) Pickling. *(2 marks)*

(b) Food spoilage can be caused by micro-organisms. Explain how high temperature treatment can extensively prolong the storage period of food while refrigeration is far less effective. *(4 marks)*

(c) Why is it inadvisable to re-freeze food which has been frozen before? *(4 marks)*

(d) Houseflies play an important part in spreading the organisms which can cause typhoid, cholera and food poisoning. State four steps that could be carried out to reduce the risk of houseflies transmitting diseases to man. *(4 marks)*

(20 marks)

QUESTION 37

(a)   The diagram shows a food web

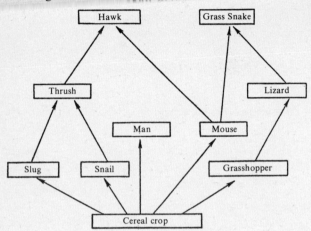

i)   Select from the food web a complete food chain consisting of **four** organisms.   *(1 mark)*

ii)   Give a named example from the food web of each of the following: a producer, a primary consumer (herbivore) and a secondary consumer (carnivore).   *(3 marks)*

iii)   What is the ultimate source of energy for this food web?   *(1 mark)*

(b)   Explain how this energy is made available to man through this food web.   *(5 marks)*

(c)   Explain what is likely to happen to the concentration of oxygen in the air surrounding the plants of a cereal crop during a 24-hour period of the growing season.   *(5 marks)*

(d)   i)   Why is the element nitrogen essential to all organisms?   *(1 mark)*

ii)   Bacteria are closely involved with the circulation of nitrogen in the environment. Briefly state the role of each of the bacteria involved.   *(4 marks)*

(Total 20 marks)

ANSWER 1

(a)

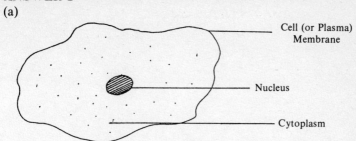

A typical animal cell as seen with a light microscope.

(b) i) A sperm cell differs from the one drawn above in that it is divided into 3 portions.

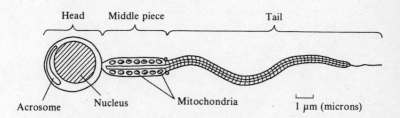

At the tip of the head, there is a small sac called the **acrosome** which contains enzymes. When released these can penetrate the cell membrane of an ovum.

The nucleus of the sperm cell contains the haploid number of chromosomes, i.e. 23.

The middle piece contains a large number of mitochondria which break down glucose to release energy (Internal Respiration) for the tail to beat.

The tail allows the sperm to swim towards the ovum.

ii) The function of a red blood cell (erythrocyte) is to transport oxygen and carbon dioxide around the body. For this purpose it has the following adaptations:—

It contains **Haemoglobin,** which is able to combine reversibly with oxygen or carbon dioxide.

It has no nucleus, this allows greater room to carry haemoglobin.

It is described as being a biconcave disc in shape. This

produces a large surface area through which gases can diffuse.

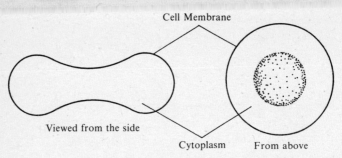

Cell Membrane

Viewed from the side

Cytoplasm   From above

iii) A sensory neurone has two large extensions of its cytoplasm, a **dendron** and an **axon.** The nucleus is contained in the cell body. The dendron conducts a nerve impulse towards the cell body, the axon conducts it away from the cell body.

The axon and dendron are surrounded by a fatty layer called the **myelin** sheath which speeds up the rate of conduction of a nerve impulse.

(c) Deoxyribonucleic acid (DNA) contains a series of stored codes for the manufacture of proteins within the cell. DNA is located in the the nucleus forming the chromosomes.

Ribonucleic Acid (RNA) is a smaller molecule[1] than DNA. It diffuses into the nucleus and makes a copy of a small part of a chromosome (DNA). It then passes out through the pores in the nuclear membrane to the ribosomes and endoplasmic reticulum where it ensures that amino acids are linked to form the correct protein.

Ribosomes. These are sites at which amino acids are linked together by **peptide** bonds to form a protein.

Mitochondria. These are the sites of internal respiration which **release energy**[2] which can be used for the formation of the peptide bond in protein synthesis.

(d) i) Liver cells are able to convert glucose to glycogen for storage.

ii) Cells in the stomach lining (oxyntic cells) are able to produce HCl.

iii) Bone forming cells (osteoblasts) secrete calcium phosphate around themselves.

iv) Rod cells found in the retina contain visual purple **(Rhodopsin).**

1. There are actually a number of types of RNA which perform different functions, e.g. messenger RNA, transfer RNA.

2. A common error made by students is to say that mitochondria "produce" or "make" energy, or to describe them as the "power stations" of the cell. These answers are too vague and may be penalised.

ANSWER 2

(a) i) An organelle is the name given to a definite structure which can be seen within the cell. Two examples would be **Mitochondria** and **Ribosomes.**

ii) Groups of cells with a similar appearance and which perform similar functions are known as tissues.

(b) i) Ciliated epithelium is found lining the inside of the nose, the respiratory passages and also the oviducts. It consists of column-shaped cells which possess tiny hairs called **cilia.** The cells are attached to a basement membrane. Mucus secreting cells are often found in this type of tissue, the beating action of the cilia cause the mucus to be transported along.

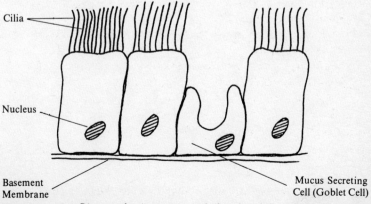

Diagram showing structure of ciliated epithelium.

ii) Compact bone has a hard white appearance and is found forming the surface layer of all bones. When examined under a microscope this type of bone can be seen to consist of **Haversian systems.** Each Haversian system consists of the following:—

a) a central Haversian canal containing blood vessels, nerves and lymph vessels.

b) **Lamellae** which are plates of bone laid down around the central Haversian canal.

c) **Lacunae** which are spaces within the bone which contain the bone cells (osteocytes).

d) **Canaliculi** which are fine channels which carry tissue fluid containing nutrients and oxygen from the Haversian canal to the bone cells (osteocytes).

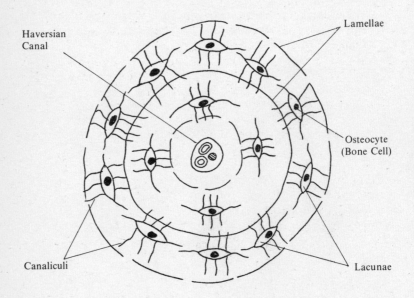

Structure of compact bone.

iii) Involuntary muscle is found in the walls of the internal organs, e.g. alimentary canal, ureters, bladder, arteries, arterioles and the uterus. It consists of sheets of separate cells, each of which contains a single nucleus.[1] The cells do not show any stripes and cannot be controlled by conscious thought. Connective tissue binds the cells together.

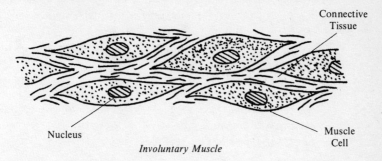

Involuntary Muscle

(c) Chromosomes are long strands of material found in the nucleus. They consist of protein and deoxyribonucleic acid (DNA). Chromosomes are normally only visible with a microscope when a cell is about to divide. Almost all cells in the body, including liver cells, contain 46 chromosomes in the nucleus. The exceptions to this are erythrocytes which have **no** nucleus and therefore **no** chromosomes and the gametes (sperm and ova) which only contain 23 chromosomes.

1. This is one of the essential differences between voluntary and involuntary muscle. Voluntary muscle consists of long muscle fibres which contain many nuclei and have a striped (or striated) appearance.

Key Words	
Organelle	Compact Bone
Mitochondria	Haversian canal
Endoplasmic Reticulum	Lamellae
Ribosome	Lacunae
Chromosome	Canaliculi
Deoxyribonucleic acid (DNA)	Erythrocyte
Tissue	Haemoglobin
Cilia	Neurone
	Axon and Dendron

ANSWER 3

(a) i) The germinative layer of the epidermis contains cells called Melanocytes. These produce the pigment **Melanin** which absorbs ultra violet light and protects the underlying organs from its harmful effects. The amount of melanin in the skin increases with exposure to ultra violet light.

ii) The sebaceous glands found in the dermis secrete **Sebum** which helps to keep the epidermis waterproof and reduces water loss from the body.

iii) The epidermis forms a continuous barrier around the body which prevents the entry of bacteria. In addition to this sebum, is a mild antiseptic and therefore inhibits the growth of bacteria on the skin surface.

iv) Rickets is a deficiency disease caused by a lack of vitamin D. The skin helps to prevent rickets by producing vitamin D in the sub cutaneous fat layer. This occurs when the skin is exposed to ultra violet light.[1]

(b) Normal body temperature is considered to be 36.9°C.[2]

(c) The regulation of body temperature is controlled by the **Hypothalamus.**

(d) Sweat produced by the sweat glands passes onto the epidermis. It takes **latent heat**[3] from the skin and evaporates. The removal of latent heat cools the skin and helps lower the body temperature.

(e) Light coloured clothes reflect much of the light and heat away from the body, whereas dark colours absorb the heat. Loose fitting clothes allow air to circulate around the skin surface which encourages the evaporation of sweat.

1. This is not to be confused with the production of Melanin, which also occurs on exposure to ultra violet light. Melanin is formed in the germinative layer of the epidermis. Vitamin D is formed by the action of ultra violet light on a substance called Ergosterol in the sub cutaneous fat layer.

2. This temperature is more correctly given as 36.9 ± 0.5°C, i.e. normal temperature ranges between 36.4°C — 37.4°C.

3. Latent heat is the heat energy needed to change a liquid (sweat) into a vapour.

ANSWER 4

(a) i) The part of the central nervous system which is responsible for controlling body temperature is the **hypothalamus.** This would receive information about the external temperature from two sources. Initially the **temperature receptors**[1] situated in the dermis of the skin would respond to the fall in temperature by relaying nerve impulses to the hypothalamus. Secondly the hypothalamus contains cells which are sensitive to the temperature of the blood. The blood flowing through the skin which is immersed in cold water will itself become cooled, and this fall in blood temperature will be sensed by the hypothalamus.

   ii) One change which could occur is shivering. When the muscles shiver, they are contracting rapidly and in doing so they release energy in the form of heat. Secondly the amount of sweat produced by the skin will be greatly reduced.[2]

(b) i) The arterioles which take blood to the skin surface dilate. This allows a greater flow of blood through the capillary loops which lie just beneath the epidermis. This process is known as **Vasodilation.**[3]

   ii) The blood temperature has been raised during the exercise. When this warm blood flows through capillary loops near the skin surface, large amounts of heat can be lost by **radiation.**

(c) i) Heat can be gained by the body from the following processes: respiration, contraction of skeletal muscles,[4] other metabolic reactions, hot food and drinks and from the environment on a hot day (any two of these could be stated). Heat can be lost from the body by the following processes: **conduction, convection, radiation, evaporation** and also via the urine, faeces and expired air (all of which are at body temperature). Again only 2 of these need be stated.

(d) i) The outer layer of the skin consists of dead cells and is known as the **cornified** (or horny) **layer.** When subjected to friction this layer is worn away but is constantly being replaced by new cells which have been produced in the germinative layer.

ii) Excretion is the removal of the waste products of the metabolic reactions of the body. The sweat produced by the skin removes large quantities of water and small quantities of urea, both of which can be classed as excretory products.

1. The temperature receptors are nerve endings found in the dermis layer of the skin, all over the body. They respond to increases or decreases in temperature by producing nerve impulses.

2. A number of other changes could have been described here, e.g. Vasoconstriction which is reduced blood flow in the capillaries near the skin surface. Alternatively contraction of the hair errector muscles (erector pili muscles) causes the hairs to stand on end (goose bumps) which traps an insulating layer of air. However this is not thought to produce a significant effect in man although it is important in animals with more hair (e.g. cats).

3. When the body temperature falls, vasoconstriction occurs and the arterioles supplying the skin constrict. A very common **error** on this question is for students to state that the blood vessels move nearer the skin surface. This is not the case, the blood vessels dilate or constrict, they **never** move up or down.

4. Heat is given as a side product of many chemical reactions in the body such as respiration or muscle contraction.

Key Words	
Epidermis	Hypothalamus
Melanocyte	Vasodilation
Melanin	Vasoconstriction
Sebaceous gland	Arterioles
Sebum	Evaporation
Rickets	Latent heat
	Radiation

ANSWER 5

(a) i)

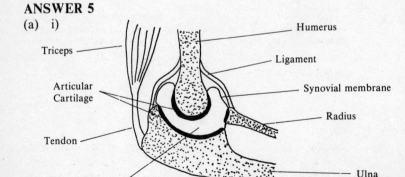

A section through the elbow joint[1]

ii) An **antagonistic pair** of muscles consists of two muscles whose actions oppose each other. In this case when one muscle contracts and shortens it will bend (flex) the elbow, this muscle is known as a **flexor**. When the other muscle contracts and shortens it will straighten (extend) the elbow and is known as an **extensor**. At the same time as the flexor is contracting, the extensor muscle is relaxing and vice versa. The muscle which acts as the extensor for the elbow is the **triceps** muscle and the flexor is the **biceps** muscle.

(b) [2]If a heavy object is lifted with the back bent and the legs straight, most of the weight will be taken by the muscles in the **lumbar** region of the back. This can result in muscle strain in this region or damage to the vertebral column such as a "slipped intervertebral disc." If the back is kept straight and the knees are bent, the strain is taken by the powerful thigh muscles which avoids the risk of damage to the back.

(c) [3]Two functions of the skeleton are:
   a) Protection, e.g. the skull protects the brain, the ribs protect the organs of the thorax.
   b) Support, e.g. the vertebral column supports the body in an upright posture.

1. This illustrates the importance of reading the question carefully. A **named** example of a **hinge** joint is required. An all too common fault in answering this question arises from carelessness in students who fail to name the joint they have drawn or simply ignore the instructions and draw other synovial joints such as a ball and socket joint.

2. With this type of general question, most people could give an answer based on their general knowledge. However, to obtain good marks for this, it is important for you to show the examiner that you possess information which a person who has not studied human biology, does not, e.g. referring to the lumbar region of the back.

3. You should always give examples of these functions.

ANSWER 6

(a) There are 3 types (or orders) of levers, the most common of these is known as the third order lever. In this case, the effort is applied between the pivot (fulcrum) and the load to be moved. An example of this can be seen at the elbow joint.

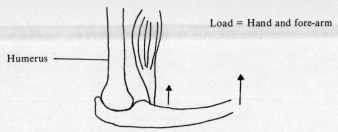

Humerus

Load = Hand and fore-arm

Fulcrum = Elbow joint

A diagram showing the elbow acting as a lever.

(b) **Ligaments** are elastic and link one bone to another. **Tendons** are non-elastic and link a muscle to a bone. The elastic property of ligaments is necessary to allow a degree of movement between bones at a joint. However, tendons must be non-elastic to transfer all the energy of muscle contraction into moving the bone.

(c) i) 1 = Spinous process
     2 = Neural canal
     3 = Transverse process
     4 = Centrum (or body)

   ii) Part 2 is the neural canal through which runs the spinal cord.

(d) **Fibrous** (fixed) joints can be found between the bones of the skull where they form the sutures.
A **cartilaginous** (slightly moveable) joint can be seen between adjacent vertebrae (and between the bones of the pelvis forming the pubic symphasis).

(e) As the body weight is pushed forwards, the muscles of the back, particularly in the lumbar region, have to contract to maintain the balance. This can lead to muscle fatigue and disorders in this region. In addition to this, the toes are pushed into the front of the shoes which can cause corns, bunions and hammer toes.

Key Words
Fibrous joint
Cartilaginous joint
Synovial joint
Ligament
Tendon

Antagonistic pair
Flexor
Extensor
Spinous process
Neural canal
Centrum

ANSWER 7

(a) [1]During the formation of urine, two main processes occur: **ultra-filtration** and **selective reabsorption.** In the description below the stages in urine formation are covered under the headings of the different parts of the nephron.

Glomerulus and Bowman's Capsule

Blood from the renal artery is under high pressure when it enters the capillaries in the **glomerulus.** This pressure causes fluid and small molecules to be forced out of the glomerulus and into the Bowman's capsule. This process is known as **ultra filtration.** The liquid collected in the Bowman's capsule is known as the **glomerular filtrate.** Red blood cells (erythrocytes) and large molecules such as **proteins** are too big to pass out of the glomerulus and so they remain in the capillary. The glomerular filtrate contains substances such as glucose, amino acids, urea, salt and water. The filtrate is similar to blood plasma but has less protein.

The Proximal (or first) coiled tubule

After the Bowman's capsule, the filtrate passes to this region of the kidney tubule where selective reabsorption begins. Glucose and amino acids are reabsorbed back into the bloodstream by active transport. The cells in this part of the tubule possess tiny projections called **microvilli.** These increase the surface area available for reabsorption. The liquid leaving the proximal (first) coiled tubule passes into the loop of Henlé.

The Loop of Henlé

As the liquid passes around the loop of Henlé both salt and water are reabsorbed into the blood capillary. This region is responsible for the greatest reabsorption of water, which occurs by **osmosis.**

Distal (or second) coiled tubule

The reabsorption of salt and water continues in this region of the tubule.

The collecting duct

Further amounts of water are absorbed from the collecting duct back into the bloodstream. The volume reabsorbed is controlled by the level of **Anti Diuretic Hormone (ADH)** in the blood. ADH is released from the pituitary gland, its effect is to make the walls of the collecting duct more permeable to water.

43

When this occurs, more water is reabsorbed into the blood and therefore less is lost in the urine.
From the collecting duct, urine drains into the pelvis of the kidney before being passed down the ureter to the bladder.

(b) i)   It would have been 140 mg per dm^3.

ii) After 20 hours, graph L reached 280 mg per dm^3 and graph M reached 40 mg per dm^3.

iii) One of the functions of the liver is to break down excess amino acids. This process is known as **de-amination**[2] and produces urea as a waste product. The urea then passes into the bloodstream. In the kidneys, urea is filtered at the glomerulus and passes out in the urine. Thus the liver produces urea and the kidneys remove it from the body.

Graph L.
After 2 hours the kidneys are removed, therefore urea is not being removed from the blood, but the liver is still producing it. So the level in the blood rises. After 8 hours, the liver is removed so no urea is being produced and as none is removed by the kidneys, the level stays constant.
Graph M.
After 2 hours, the liver is removed so no more urea is being produced. However the kidneys are still removing it from the blood, therefore the level falls. After 8 hours, the kidneys are removed so no urea is being removed or produced and the level stays constant.

1. In an essay type question such as this, it is important to construct a plan before beginning. In this case, it is most convenient to use different parts of the nephron as headings, e.g.
    a. Glomerulus and Bowman's capsule — filtration.
    b. Proximal coiled tubule — amino acids, glucose, active transport.
    c. Loop of Henlé — salt, water, osmosis.
    d. Distal coiled tubule — salt, water.
    e. Collecting duct — water, ADH.

2. De-amination of amino acids and the production of urea is a favourite topic for an examination question. In this process, amino acids are split into a nitrogen containing part which is converted to urea. The residue is then converted to glycogen for storage or is broken down during internal respiration.

ANSWER 8

(a) i)   Structures labelled A are **Microvilli.** These projections of the cytoplasm increase the surface area available for reabsorption.[1]

     ii) These thin walls provide a very short distance over which diffusion has to occur.

     iii) Structures B are **Mitochondria.** They are the site of internal respiration and release the energy needed for active reabsorption.[2]

(b) i)   As the filtrate passes around the tubule, water is reabsorbed by osmosis back into the bloodstream. Most water is reabsorbed from the loop of Henlé. The remainder from the distal (second) coiled tubule and the collecting duct. The volume of water reabsorbed from the collecting duct is controlled by Anti Diuretic Hormone.[3]

     ii) Glucose and amino acids are filtered at the glomerulus but are then completely reabsorbed, so they do not appear in the urine.

     iii) Proteins are present in blood plasma but not in the glomerular filtrate or the urine. This is because protein molecules are too large to be forced through the capillary walls in the glomerulus. The protein molecules remain in the bloodstream.

(c) i)   In hot weather, large volumes of water are lost from the skin by sweating, therefore there is less to be excreted in the urine. In cold weather, less sweating occurs and a greater volume of water must be lost in the urine.

     ii) **Urea** is the principal nitrogenous compound present in urine. In cold weather, large volumes of water are present in the urine, which dilutes the urea, lowering its concentration. In warm weather, the urea concentration is higher due to the reduced volume of water present.

(d) A reflex action is caused by a stimulus which produces a response and does not involve the conscious control of the brain. In the case of micturition, the stimulus is the presence of urine in the bladder and the response is the relaxation of the sphincter muscle at the base of the bladder, allowing urine to leave through the urethra.

1. Microvilli are also found located on the villi in the small intestine.

2. Glucose and amino acids are reabsorbed by active transport, i.e. against a concentration gradient.

3. ADH is released into the blood from the posterior lobe of the pituitary gland. In the presence of ADH, the walls of the collecting duct become more permeable to water. Thus more water passes from the collecting duct into the blood and less is lost in the urine.

Key Words	Osmosis
Excretion	Nephron
Urea	Glomerulus
De-amination	Loop of Henlé
Micturition	

ANSWER 9

(a) i) Air is drawn into the lungs by the following mechanism: The diaphragm contracts and becomes flattened. The intercostal muscles contract and lift the rib cage upwards and outwards. Both of these changes increase the volume inside the thorax. As the thorax is airtight, this causes the pressure inside to drop. Thus the pressure on the outside of the lungs is reduced and is now less than atmospheric pressure. Air is therefore drawn in and inflates the lungs.

(b) i) Tissue respiration is the process by which simple food molecules are broken down to release energy. This occurs in the mitochondria of all cells and the waste products are carbon dioxide, and water. (Tissue respiration is also known as cell respiration or internal respiration).

ii) The energy released in tissue respiration is used to form a chemical called **Adenosine Triphosphate (ATP).** This is produced when a phosphate group is chemically linked to a substance called **Adenosine Diphosphate (ADP).**[1]

Adenosine—P—P + P —Energy→ Adenosine—P—P—P

Adenosine diphosphate + phosphate + energy ⟶ Adenosine Triphosphate.

ATP acts as an energy storage substance. It diffuses from the mitochondria to whichever part of the cell needs energy.

Once there, ATP breaks down and makes the energy available for any cell processes requiring it.

(c) i) The usual amount of carbon dioxide in the air is 0.04%.

ii) After inspiring increasing amounts of carbon dioxide, the breathing rate and tidal volume both increased.

iii) Volume of air per minute = Tidal volume x Breathing rate.

For 0.04% CO_2
Volume of air per min = 520 x 14 cm^3/min
= 7,280 cm^3/min

For 6.00% CO_2
Volume of air per min = 2100 x 28
= 58,800 cm^3/min

iv) [2]To calculate — volume of oxygen being used by the body when breathing 0.04% CO_2.
Given:
(from part iii) above) Volume of air taken in = 7,280 cm^3 per minute.
Of this 20% is oxygen.
Only 20% of oxygen taken in is used.

Volume of oxygen breathed in per minute is 20% of 7,280 cm^3.
= $\dfrac{20}{100}$ x 7280
= 1456 cm^3 of 0_2 per minute.
Volume of oxygen used per minute is 20% of 1456 cm^3.
= $\dfrac{20}{100}$ x 1456
= 291.2 cm^3 of oxygen per minute.
Thus 291.2 cm^3 of oxygen is used by the body each minute.

(d) The **medulla oblongata** contains the respiratory centre which controls breathing rate and tidal volume. It is sensitive to the levels of carbon dioxide in the blood.

---

1. In general, when a chemical link is formed, energy must be supplied, e.g. to convert ADP and P into ATP. The opposite occurs when a chemical link is broken, energy is released. (The correct chemical symbol for a phosphate group is PO_4 not simply P).

2. Whenever attempting a calculation question, it is vital that you set your work out neatly and in explained steps. It is often helpful to start off by simply stating the information given and the factor to be calculated. Although you will not directly gain marks for this, it does frequently help to simplify the question and enable you to see the basic calculation required. Throughout the calculation you should ensure that you have used the **correct units,** e.g. cm^3 or cm^3 per min in this case. At the end of the question check your answer to see if it is in the right units, e.g. cm^3 of oxygen per minute and see if it is the right order of magnitude, i.e. nearly 300, not 30 or 3000.

ANSWER 10

(a) i)   Letter C represents the inspiratory reserve volume, it has a value of 3000 cm^3.

ii) Letter E represents the vital capacity which has a value of 4,500 cm^3.

iii) The residual volume is represented by letter A and has a value of 1,500 cm^3. [1].

(b) i)   Tidal volume is the volume of air breathed in or out during normal quiet breathing.

ii) Oxygen and carbon dioxide are exchanged between the blood and inspired air in the **alveoli.** Around 150 cm^3 of air inspired does not reach the alveoli but remains in the trachea, bronchi and bronchioles. This is known as the **dead space,** because the air in this region is then expired without any exchange of gases.

(c) **Apparatus**

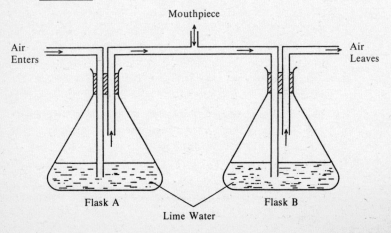

Method

The apparatus should be set up as above. The subject pinches his nose and then breathes in and out through the mouthpiece. Air is drawn in through the limewater in flask A. When the subject breathes in and passes out through the limewater in flask B when the subject breathes out.

Results

The expected result would be that the limewater in flask A would remain clear but the limewater in flask B would turn cloudy. This result would show that there is a greater concentration of carbon dioxide in expired air than inspired air.

(d) Oxygen and carbon dioxide pass through the wall of the alveoli by diffusion. The following adaptations allow diffusion to take place very rapidly.

    i) The internal surface of the alveoli are lined with moisture to allow gas molecules to dissolve.

    ii) The alveoli walls are only one cell thick, which produces a very short distance for diffusion to occur across.

    iii) Each alveolus is surrounded by blood capillaries and therefore receives a rich blood supply.[2]

1.   Letter B represents the tidal volume and letter D the expiratory reserve volume.

2.   The rounded shape of the alveolus also increases the surface area available for diffusion.

ANSWER 11

(1) i) When the rubber sheet is pulled down, the **volume** inside the bell jar is **increased.** As the bell jar is completely airtight, the **pressure** inside the jar is **reduced.** Thus the pressure on the outside of the balloons is now lower than atmospheric pressure. A small amount of air is drawn in, causing the balloons to inflate slightly.

    ii) Letter A represents the trachea.
Letter B represents the bronchus.
Letter C represents the thoracic wall (the ribs and intercostal muscles).
Letter D represents the thoracic cavity.
Letter E represents the diaphragm.

iii) 1. The rubber sheet is a poor model of the diaphragm because for this apparatus to work it must be pulled downwards. In the body the diaphragm never curves downwards, even when it is contracted.

2. The lungs fill the chest cavity in the body. The balloons are too small in proportion to the size of the bell jar to illustrate this.

3. During inspiration and expiration the rib cage moves up and down, in and out. The glass sides of the bell jar are unable to show this.

4. The lungs cannot be compared to balloons because they contain small tubes called bronchioles and millions of air sacs called alveoli.

5. The outside of the lungs and the inside of the thoracic cavity are covered by the pleural membranes. This model does not have anything to represent these membranes.

(b) **Anaerobic respiration** is the breakdown of simple food molecules (usually glucose) to release energy in the absence of oxygen. This type of respiration takes place in the muscles when there is a shortage of oxygen caused by strenuous exercise. During anaerobic respiration in the muscles lactic acid is produced.

(c) At the end of exercise a person continues to breathe heavily for some time. This occurs so that extra oxygen is carried in the blood to the muscles. The oxygen is used to remove **lactic acid** which has built up during exercise in the muscles. The heavy breathing to provide oxygen to remove lactic acid after exercise has finished is known as **repaying the oxygen debt.**

ANSWER 12

(a) There are approximately 300 million alveoli in the lungs and their function is to provide a site for the exchange of carbon dioxide and oxygen. Each alveolus is surrounded by a network of blood capillaries. Blood has been brought to these capillaries from the **pulmonary artery** and eventually leaves the lungs by the **pulmonary vein.**

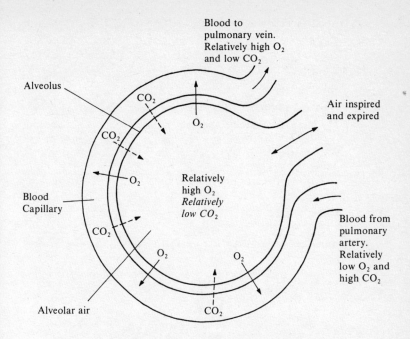

Diagram showing gas exchange in an alveolus.

Blood entering the capillary around the alveolus has relatively little oxygen and a relatively high level of carbon dioxide. However, air in the alveolus has relatively more oxygen and less carbon dioxide. Thus there is a **concentration gradient** between the alveolar air and the blood in the capillary. Therefore oxygen diffuses from the alveolus into the blood capillary and carbon dioxide diffuses from the blood capillary into the alveolus (see diagram above).

Thus the blood leaving the lungs now has a relatively high concentration of oxygen and a low concentration of carbon dioxide.

(b) [1]

Pulmonary Artery	Pulmonary Vein
1. Contains higher concentration of carbon dioxide.	Lower concentration carbon dioxide.
2. Contains lower concentration of oxygen.	Higher concentration of oxygen.

(c) i) The tidal volume and ventilation rate will both increase.

ii) Regular strenuous exercise produces a variety of effects on breathing.
   (1) The person's vital capacity is increased (their lungs can hold more air).
   (2) The number of blood capillaries in the lungs may also increase. So they can supply more oxygen to the blood.
   (3) Breathing during exercise is more regular and controlled. It is also easier due to relaxation of smooth muscle in the bronchioles which increases their diameter.

(d) Cigarette smoking is closely associated with the following conditions:—
   1. Lung cancer — caused by chemicals inhaled through smoking.
   2. Heart disease — cigarettes release **carbon monoxide** which combines with haemoglobin in erythrocytes. This increases the risk of heart attacks.
   3. Chronic bronchitis (inflammation of the trachea and bronchi). This is often associated with emphysema, which is a condition where the walls of the alveoli break down, leaving the sufferer short of breath.
   4. Raised blood pressure — nicotine is a stimulant drug.
   5. Smoking in pregnancy can produce premature and under-weight babies.

There are a number of other conditions which may be associated with cigarette smoking, but those listed above are amongst the most common.

1. When asked to state differences in a question of this nature, it is useful to put your answer in table form.

Key Words	
Respiration	Alveoli
Aerobic	Diffusion
Anaerobic	Tidal volume
Adenosine Triphosphate (ATP)	Vital capacity
Adenosine Diphosphate (ADP)	Residual volume
Lactic Acid	Reserve volumes
Oxygen debt	Dead space

ANSWER 13

(a) i) The total amount of energy released by the oxidation of foods was
$3540 + 2390 + 1880 = 7,810$ kJ.[1]
The total amount of energy lost in the same time was
$9,800 + 380 = 10,180$ kJ.
Thus the amount of energy which must be made up from food reserves is 2,370 kJ (7,810 − 10,180 kJ).

ii) This energy can be made up by the breakdown of fat stored under the skin or the breakdown of **glycogen** stored in the liver and muscles.

(b) i) Fluoride is added to the water supply to help prevent tooth decay. This mineral becomes absorbed by the enamel and dentine of the tooth which then becomes harder and more resistant to attack by acids.

ii) Vitamin D can be obtained from two sources: the diet and also the skin. When the skin is exposed to ultra violet light, it is able to produce Vitamin D in the sub cutaneous fat layer. Thus a person who is exposed to large amounts of sunlight will require less dietary vitamin D, than a person who receives very little sunlight.

iii) Fresh vegetables and fruits are some of the best sources of the vitamins which are essential for health. For example citrus fruits provide Vitamin C and green salads can provide Vitamins A, B_2, and K.

iv) Roughage is the name given to the parts of the diet which pass through the body undigested. It is composed of mainly cellulose fibres from plant cell walls. It is important in the diet as it adds bulk to the faeces and stimulates peristalsis (contractions) in the colon. Lack of roughage may lead to constipation.

(c) A **balanced diet** is one which provides all of the items listed below in the correct proportions:—
1. Protein
2. Carbohydrate
3. Fat
4. Vitamins

5. Minerals
6. Roughage
7. Water

1. Whenever using figures it is essential that you also state the **units** (i.e. kJ in this case). Otherwise your answer is meaningless and marks will be lost.

ANSWER 14

(a) i) Tube 1 acts as **a control,** showing that [1]hydrogen peroxide alone does not release enough oxygen to relight the glowing splint.

ii) Manganese dioxide is a chemical **catalyst**[2] which is causing hydrogen peroxide to break down and release oxygen.

iii) Both fresh liver and fresh blood contain **enzymes** which are biological catalysts — made of protein. These enzymes cause the hydrogen peroxide to break down and release oxygen.

iv) One of the properties of enzymes is that when heated above 60°C they become permanently changed or **denatured.**[3] Once they have been denatured they no longer function, even if they are cooled. After boiling liver and blood, the enzymes they contain will have been denatured and therefore they are unable to catalyse the breakdown of hydrogen peroxide. This explains why no oxygen is released from tubes 5 and 7.

v) Manganese dioxide is a chemical catalyst which is not made of protein. Therefore boiling this substance does not produce any change in its action as a catalyst.

vi) Two factors which must be kept constant are the **temperature** and the **pH** of the tubes.[3]

(b) i)

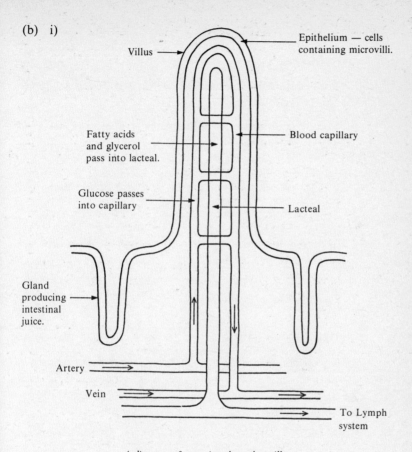

A diagram of a section through a villus.

ii) Fatty acids and glycerol are absorbed by the epithelial cells of the villus and then passed into the **lacteal** (lymph capillary). Glucose is also absorbed by the epithelium of the villus but is then passed into the blood capillary. All of these substances are absorbed by active transport.

1. Hydrogen peroxide does decompose on its own to release oxygen. This process however is very slow and a catalyst is needed to release enough oxygen to relight a glowing splint.

2. A catalyst is a substance which changes the rate of a chemical reaction. It does not take part in the reaction and is unchanged by it.

3. General properties of proteins and enzymes in particular are that they are affected by heat and pH (acidity or alkalinity).

ANSWER 15

(a) i) Hepatic artery originates from the aorta and terminates in the liver.

ii) The hepatic vein originates in the liver and terminates in the inferior vena cava.

iii) The hepatic portal vein originates in the intestines and terminates in the liver.

(b) [1]

Hepatic Artery	Hepatic Vein
1. Relatively high concentration of oxygen.	Lower oxygen concentration.
2. Relatively low carbon dioxide concentration.	Higher carbon dioxide concentration.
[2] 3. Lower concentration of urea.	Higher concentration of urea.

(c) [1]

Hepatic Portal Vein	Hepatic Vein
1. Higher concentration of glucose.	Lower concentration of glucose.
2. Higher concentration of amino acids.	Lower concentration of amino acids.
[2] 3. Lower concentration of urea.	Higher concentration of urea.

(d) The hepatic portal veins start off as capillaries in one organ of the body (intestines) and terminates as capillaries in another organ (the liver).

(e) i) The pancreas releases pancreatic juice into the duodenum and the liver produces **bile** which is released from the **gall bladder** into the **duodenum**.

ii) **Bile** does not contain any enzymes[3] but it contains salts which **emulsify** fats, i.e. break them up into tiny droplets. Once the fats have been emulsified, they have a much greater surface area for enzymes to act upon.

Pancreatic juice contains the enzyme **Lipase** which breaks down fats into fatty acids and glycerol.

1. Both of these questions can be answered most concisely if tables are used. Furthermore, both questions ask for differences in **chemical** composition of blood. Differences in pressure or flow of blood will gain no marks.

2. See question 7 for the relationship between the liver and urea.

3. A common mistake made by students is to claim that there are enzymes in bile juice. This is totally incorrect.

ANSWER 16

(a) [1]A piece of lean meat is composed of mainly protein. The digestion of this meat can be divided into stages according to the different parts of the alimentary canal.

In the mouth

Initially the meat will be chewed in the mouth by the molars and premolars. This **mechanical digestion** will increase the surface area for the action of enzymes on the meat. Also in the mouth, the meat will have been lubricated with saliva and then swallowed.

The stomach

After being passed down the oesophagus by peristalsis the meat will arrive in the stomach. Here it will be acted upon by two substances, **hydrochloric acid** and the enzyme **pepsin (gastric protease).** Hydrochloric acid begins to break down the meat into peptides and amino acids. The acid also provides the optimum conditions for the enzyme pepsin (gastric protease) to function. Pepsin (gastric protease) acts on the protein in the meat in the following way:—

$$\text{Protein} \xrightarrow[\text{(Gastric protease)}]{\text{Pepsin}} \text{peptides (or peptones)}$$

When it is suitably digested, food is released from the stomach by the relaxation of the pyloric sphincter.

In Duodenum

Pancreatic juice in the duodenum contains sodium hydrogen carbonate which neutralises the acid that has been produced in the stomach. This also produces the optimum pH for the enzymes which act in the duodenum. Pancreatic juice contains **Trypsinogen,** which is an inactive enzyme. This is converted to the active form **Trypsin,** by the action of an enzyme secreted by the walls of the duodenum known as **Enterokinase.**

$$\text{Trypsinogen} \xrightarrow{\text{Enterokinase}} \text{Trypsin}$$

Trypsin breaks down proteins and peptides into amino acids.

In the small Intestine

The juices secreted by the walls of the small intestine contain a mixture of protein digesting enzymes (peptidases) which are given the collective name **Erepsin.** Erepsin completes the digestion of the meat protein by breaking down any remaining **peptides** into **amino acids.**

Thus in summary, the following enzymes are involved in the different stages for digestion of meat proteins.

1. **Pepsin** (Gastric protease)
2. **Trypsin(ogen)** and **Enterokinase**
3. **Erepsin**

(b) **Peristalsis** is the name given to the waves of muscular contraction which move food along the alimentary canal.

All parts of the alimentary canal contain two types of muscle fibres, circular and longitudinal. The muscle types are antagonistic to each other, i.e. when one contracts the other relaxes. The diagram below illustrates how peristalsis causes food to be moved along:—

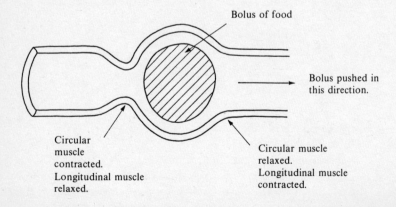

Diagram showing peristalsis.

1. Before starting a question such as this it is important to do a short plan of what you intend to write, e.g.

Stages:
1. Mouth — Mastication (chewing) — mechanical digestion.
2. Stomach — Hydrochloric acid, pepsin.
3. Duodenum — Enterokinase, trypsinogen.
4. Intestine — Erepsin.

This helps to keep your answer concise.

Key Words	
Digestion	Enzyme
Balanced Diet	Denaturation
Vitamin	Protease
Mineral	Lipase
Roughage	Hepatic artery
Villus	Hepatic vein
Lacteal	Hepatic portal vein
Peristalsis	Bile
Catalyst	Emulsification
	Gall bladder

ANSWER 17

(a) i) There are a number of different types of white blood cell found in the body. These include **lymphocytes** and **granulocytes.** Lymphocytes are produced by lymph nodes and other lymphatic tissue, and their function is to produce **antibodies.**

Granulocytes are found in larger numbers than lymphocytes and are produced in the **bone marrow.** They are slightly larger than lymphocytes and have a very distinctive nucleus, which is divided up into a number of lobes. Granulocytes help to protect the body from infection by engulfing microbes (a process called **phagocytosis**).[1]

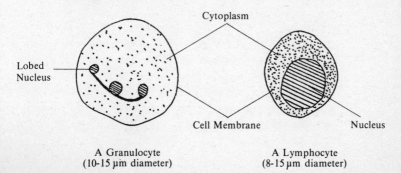

Cytoplasm

Lobed Nucleus

Cell Membrane

Nucleus

A Granulocyte
(10-15 μm diameter)

A Lymphocyte
(8-15 μm diameter)

ii) When a foreign material enters the body, the immediate response is the production of a substance which will cause it to become harmless. The foreign material is called the **Antigen** and the substances produced in response are called **Antibodies.** Thus antibodies are a group of substances (proteins) which are produced by lymphocytes and other cells to destroy or render harmless "foreign" chemicals, tissues or invading microbes in the body.

Antigens are "foreign" chemicals, tissues or micro-organisms which cause the production of antibodies. Examples of antigens are drugs such as penicillin, organ transplants or bacteria.

iii) To prevent a subject catching a particular disease, e.g. tuberculosis or measles, immunity can be produced by injecting them with a **vaccine.** The vaccine contains a sample of micro-organisms which cause the person to produce antibodies against that particular disease. The micro-organisms in the vaccine may be a very dilute sample of the disease causing micro-organism or even a sample of killed micro-organisms. However the body still recognises the microbe and begins to produce antibodies against it.

The injection of a **serum** can also be used to prevent infection but more frequently it is used to treat an infection which may have already occurred, e.g. rabies or tetanus. Serum is the name given to the part of the blood which remains after the cells and clotting proteins have been removed. Thus if serum is obtained from another person or animal which has been in contact with the disease, it will be rich in antibodies to fight the micro-organism involved.

In summary:

1. An injection of a vaccine causes the subject to produce their **own antibodies.**[2] This provides long term immunity.

2. An injection of a serum gives the subject an immediate dose of antibodies to fight the infection. As the subject has not made the antibodies himself[3], this type of immunity is short lived.

(b) The lymphatic system is closely associated with the circulatory system and has a number of functions, such as:
1. It provides a root for returning excess tissue fluid to the blood system.
2. It is involved with the absorption of fats from the intestines and their transport around the body.[4]

1. Phagocytosis is another common examination topic. You should be able to draw fully labelled diagrams illustrating this process.

2. This is an example of **artificial active immunity.**

3. This is an example of **artificial passive immunity.**

4. See question 14(b).

ANSWER 18

(a) i) Blood can be divided into different groups according to which type of proteins are present on the surface of the red cells. These protein "markers" are known as **Agglutinogens (antigens)** and there are two types, called A or B. The different blood groups are shown below.

Group	Agglutinogen on red cells
A	A
B	B
AB	both A and B
O	Neither A or B

In addition to the agglutinogen present on the red cells, the different groups contain **agglutinins (antibodies)** occuring in the plasma. These agglutinins cause agglutination[1] of red cells of other groups. Thus the agglutinogens and agglutinins present in the four blood groups are shown in the following table:—

Group	Agglutinogen (antigen) on red cells	Agglutinins (antibodies) in plasma
A	A	anti B
B	B	anti A
AB	Both A and B	neither anti A or anti B
O	neither A or B	Both anti A and anti B

ii) **Serum** from group A blood will contain anti B agglutinins and serum from group B blood will contain anti A agglutinins. If a few drops from the sample of unknown blood were added to group A serum and group B serum separately, the results would show which group the unknown blood belonged to. For example, if the blood did not agglutinate when added to group A serum but did with group B serum, these would indicate that the blood was group A. The possible results that could be obtained are shown in the table below:—

Group A serum	Group B serum	Blood group of sample
X	✓	A
✓	X	B
✓	✓	AB
X	X	O

Where X shows no agglutination occured and
✓ shows agglutination did occur.

(b) i)

Arteries	Veins
1. Thick muscular walls.	Relatively thinner walls which contain no muscle tissue.
2. Relatively small lumen.	Relatively large lumen.
3. Do not possess valves.	Large veins possess valves.

(c) Liver ⎯⎯⎯⎯⎯⟶
   1. Hepatic vein
   2. Vena cava
   3. Right atrium
   4. Right ventricle
   5. Pulmonary artery (to lungs)
   6. Pulmonary vein
   7. Left atrium
   8. Left ventricle
   9. Aorta
  10. Renal artery to the kidney

1. A common mistake is to use the word "clotting", when referring to the reaction between agglutinins and agglutinogens. This is incorrect, the correct term is **agglutination** or **"clumping"**.

ANSWER 19

(a) i)

Vessel	Name	oxygenated/ deoxygenated
1.	Vena cava	deoxygenated
2.	Aorta	oxygenated
3.	Pulmonary artery	deoxygenated[1]
4.	Pulmonary veins	oxygenated[2]

ii) The vessels labelled 5 are the **coronary arteries,** their function is to supply blood to the muscle of the heart. They provide nutrients and oxygen to the cardiac muscle, without which the muscle fibres would begin to die (this would produce a heart attack).

iii) The sequence of events can be described in the following stages:—
   1. While the atrium is relaxed, blood enters from the **vena cava.**
   2. As the atrium fills with blood, the pressure causes the **tricuspid** (mitral or atrioventricular) valve to be pushed **open** and blood flows into the ventricle.
   3. The atrium then contracts, forcing more blood into the ventricle.

4. The ventricle begins to contract, causing the **tricuspid valve** to **close,** preventing the backflow of blood into the atrium. At the same time the semilunar valve in the pulmonary artery is forced open.

5. As the ventricle continues to contract, blood is forced out through the **pulmonary artery,** up towards the lungs.

(b) Blood clotting takes place in the following stages:—

1. Damaged tissues and platelets release **Thrombokinase** (Thromboplastin).

2. Thrombokinase acts on prothrombin, which is an inactive enzyme present in the blood. **Prothrombin** is converted to **Thrombin.**

3. This in turn acts upon the inactive protein **Fibrinogen** converting it to **Fibrin.**

4. A mesh of fibrin forms across the wound, trapping blood cells and platelets to form a clot.

5. The clot then dries and shrinks to form a scab, which protects the tissues below while repair takes place.
For the process above to occur, calcium ions must also be present at each stage.

1. The pulmonary artery divides in two, one vessel passing to each lung.

2. There are four pulmonary veins emptying into the left atrium, two from each lung.

ANSWER 20

(a) i) Blood has two main functions, it provides the transport system of the body and is also involved with the body's defences. The main components which blood transports around the body are:—

1. **Respiratory gases** — both oxygen and carbon dioxide, are carried by the haemoglobin contained in erythrocytes (red cells).

2. **Nutrients** — the blood contains all the nutrients required by the body cells, e.g. amino acids, glucose, vitamins, minerals.

3. **Excretory products** — as well as carbon dioxide, other waste products are transported by the blood, e.g. urea.

4. **Hormones** — the endocrine glands release their products into the bloodstream, e.g. adrenaline, oestrogen.

5. **Heat** — most heat is produced by the liver and muscles. Blood collects heat from these regions of the body and then circulates to all other parts.

Blood is closely associated with the body's defence system in that it contains the white blood cells (leucocytes). These engulf bacteria and viruses or produce antibodies.[1] In addition to this, when a break in a blood vessel occurs, a clot is formed to prevent the entry of micro-organisms and thus preventing infection.

(b) i) There are a number of different valves found in the circulatory system, they have the following functions:—

1. **The Atrioventricular**[2] (mitral, or tricuspid and bicuspid) valves — these are found on both sides of the heart. They separate the atria from the ventricles. Their function is to prevent the backflow of blood into the atria when the ventricles contract.

2. **The Semilunar Valves** — these are found in the pulmonary artery and the aorta, where these vessels leave the heart. Their function is to prevent the backflow of blood into the ventricles, when the ventricles relax (i.e. during **diastole).**

3. Finally valves can be found in the large veins of the body. Their function is to ensure that blood can only travel in one direction, i.e. back towards the heart.

ii) Blood flow is maintained through veins by the following:—

1. The remaining pressure from the heart beat.[3]

2. The presence of valves which ensure blood may only flow in one direction.

3. The action of contracting muscles, pushing on the walls of the vein. Many of the large veins run through groups of voluntary muscles. When a muscle contracts, it becomes shorter and fatter. This causes the muscles to push on the side of the vein. The presence of valves in the vein result in blood being gently pushed along by the action of these muscles.

iii) The heart sounds are produced by the shutting of the two sets of heart valves. The "lubb" sound results from the closing of the atrioventricular (mitral, tricuspid and bicuspid) valves. The "dupp" sound is due to the closing of the semilunar valves in the pulmonary artery and aorta.

1. See question 17.

2. A common error when writing about the heart valves, is for students to state the valves contract and relax. This is completely incorrect, they are not composed of muscle but can be thought of as being flaps of skin.

3. After blood has flowed through the arterioles and capillaries, most of the pressure created by the heart beat has been lost.

Key Words	
Erythrocytes	Clotting (coagulation)
Lymphocytes	Artery
Granulocytes (phagocyte, polymorphonucleocyte)	Arteriole
Platelets (thrombocytes)	Vein
Phagocytosis	Capillary
Immunity (artificial/natural, active/passive)	Atrium
Serum	Ventricle
Antigen	Bicuspid valve
Antibody	Tricuspid valve
Agglutinogen	Semilunar valve
Agglutinin	Diastole
Agglutination	Systole

ANSWER 21

(a)　i)　A **reflex** is a rapid, involuntary response to a stimulus, which does not require the participation of the conscious part of the brain.

　　ii)　[1]A complete reflex action such as the withdrawal of the hand from a hot object requires a complete **reflex arc,** as illustrated below.

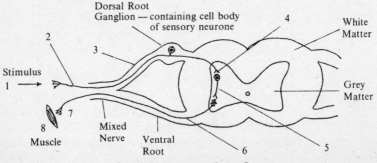

Diagram showing a complete reflex arc.
(The numbers correspond with the notes below)

1. The hot object stimulates a pain receptor in the skin which produces a nerve impulse.
2. The **nerve impulse** is transmitted along the **sensory neurone.**
3. The sensory neurone enters the spinal cord through the **dorsal root.**
4. The impulse is passed across a **synapse**[2] in the grey matter of the spinal cord to a connector neurone.
5. The **connector neurone** carries the impulse through the **grey matter** and passes it across a synapse to a motor neurone.
6. The **motor neurone** carries the impulse out of the spinal cord through the **ventral root.**
7. The motor neurone conducts the nerve impulse to the muscle.
8. The impulse crosses the **motor end plate**[3] and causes contraction of the muscle, which results in the hand being withdrawn from the hot object.

iii) If the person had consumed a quantity of **alcohol,** their response would have been much slower as alcohol depresses the activity of the nervous system.

(b) i) <u>Part A</u> is the **cerebellum** and is responsible for controlling posture, balance of muscular co-ordination.
<u>Part B</u> is the **cerebral cortex,** this has many functions including control of all voluntary movement and receiving nerve impulses from all of the sense organs in the body.
<u>Part C</u> is the **medulla oblongata** which controls many of the the body's internal processes such as breathing, heart rate, and swallowing.
<u>Part D</u> is the **hypothalamus** which controls processes such as, body temperature, blood sugar level and salt/water balance of the body fluids.

ii) <u>Part E</u> is the **pituitary gland.**

iii) The **grey matter** of the nervous system consists of the cell bodies of neurones (which includes the nuclei) and blood vessels. The white matter consists mainly of nerve fibres (i.e. axons and dendrons). Many of these are surrounded by a fatty layer called the **myelin sheath** which has a white appearance.

1. In a question of this nature a diagram can be used to help illustrate and clarify your answer. However, the question specifically asks you to **describe** the reflex and therefore a diagram alone would be insufficient.

2. A synapse is a connection between neurones which allows an impulse to pass from one neurone to another. There is a minute gap between the neurones. This is crossed by a chemical released from the ends of the neurone when a nerve impulse arrives.

3. A motor end plate is the connection between a neurone and a muscle fibre. It is very similar to a synapse.
    General point: A common error is to state that nerves or neurones carry "messages". This is incorrect, they **conduct nerve impulses.** Any reference to "messages" may result in your answer being penalised.

ANSWER 22

(a)   i)   Part A is the cornea.
           B is the lens.
           C is the retina.
           D is the optic nerve.
           E is the iris.
           F is the pupil.

      ii) The **cornea** (A) has two main functions, to protect the eye from damage and to refract rays of light onto the lens. The function of the **lens** (B) is to further refract rays of light, bringing them to a clear focus on the retina. The **retina** (C) contains the light sensitive cells called **rods** and **cones**. The nerve impulses produced by rod and cone cells in the retina are then conducted to the cerebral cortex by the optic nerve (D).

      iii) In bright sunlight the **pupil** is constricted but as a person moves into the shade the size of the pupil increases. This is brought about by contraction of the **radial** muscles and relaxation of the **circular** muscles in the **iris**.

      iv) The dilation of the pupil in dim light increases the amount of light which can enter the eye and therefore allows a clearer image to be seen.

(b)   [1]The ability of the eye to focus on objects at different distances is known as **accommodation**. When viewing a near object, the rays of light **diverge** (or spread out). This means that to refract these rays onto the retina the lens must be very **convex**. The eye ensures that the lens is convex by the following changes:—

1. The **ciliary muscles** contract inwards overcoming the pressure exerted by the vitreous humour.
2. The tension in the **suspensory ligaments** is therefore reduced.
3. The lens is relaxed and takes up its natural rounded (convex) shape.
4. The rays of light pass through the lens and are brought to a sharp focus on the retina.

(c) By possessing two eyes which have overlapping fields of view, this allows us to see objects in three dimensions. It is also important for the judgement of distances and helps to remove the blind spot effect.

1. This is a question which students frequently misunderstand or become confused about. It is important to remember that the ciliary muscle is a **ring** of muscle, which when it contracts allows the **lens to relax.** Other common mistakes are to confuse the ciliary muscle with the muscles in the iris (circular and radial) or to state that the suspensory ligaments contract and relax (they are not muscles or elastic tissue but are cord like structures).

ANSWER 23

(a) i)[1]

Rays refracted
by cornea
and lens

Light rays diverging

Near object

Rays brought to a focus behind retina

Image formation in a person with long sight (hypermetropia)

ii) This condition can be corrected by using a convex (converging) lens.

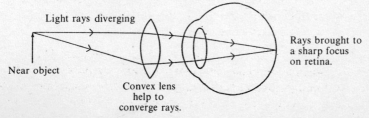

Light rays diverging

Near object

Rays brought to a sharp focus on retina.

Convex lens help to converge rays.

(b) i) A^2

    ii) A

    iii) B

(c) i)   There are two types of light sensitive cells in the **retina, rods** and **cones.** The cone cells are used to distinguish colours and fine detail and are only able to function in **high light intensities.** Thus in dim light the cones are unable to function and therefore colours cannot be seen.
Rod cells require much **lower light intensities** than cone cells. Therefore we are able to see the general shape of an object in conditions of low light. However, rod cells are unable to distinguish between the different colours (wavelengths) of light. Thus in poor light we can see the shape but not the colour of an object.

    ii) When an object is looked at directly it is focused onto a region of the retina called the **fovea (or yellow spot).** This region contains many millions of cone cells but very few rod cells. If the image of a dim object is focused onto the fovea, there will be insufficient light to stimulate the cone cells to function. Therefore the object may not be seen. However, the majority of rod cells are found around the **sides** of the retina. If the dim object is not looked at directly, the image falls on the sides of the retina and there will be sufficient light for the rod cells to be stimulated, allowing the object to be seen.

1. Most marks are lost on a question of this nature by students neglecting to **label their diagrams.** The number of marks awarded are an indication of roughly how many labels are required.

2. When light falls on a cone cell this causes the pigment **rhodopsin (visual purple)** to break down into retinene (vitamin A compound) and opsin (A protein). Retinene then stimulates a nerve impulse. To reform rhodopsin, energy must be supplied, thus ATP is needed. (See Q.9 (b)ii)).

ANSWER 24

(a) The **ossicles** are the bones of the middle ear, the **malleus** (hammer), **incus** (anvil) and **stapes** (stirrup). Their function is to transmit and amplify sound waves from the tympanic membrane (ear drum) to the oval window of the cochlea.

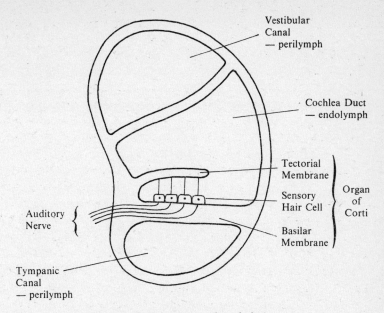

Diagram representing a section through the inner ear.

(b) The diagram above represents the structure of the **cochlea**. It can be seen to consist of three fluid filled canals. The vestibular and tympanic canals contain the fluid, **perilymph** and the cochlea duct contains **endolymph**. The cochlea duct contains a group of sensory cells which possess minute hairs. These hairs are embedded in the tectorial membrane. This structure is known as the **organ of Corti**.

The oval window covers the point where the vestibular canal comes in contact with the air filled middle ear. As the oval window vibrates, the following effects are produced:—

1. Pressure waves (vibrations) are set up in the **perilymph** of the **vestibular canal**.

2. These pressure waves are conducted through to the **endolymph** in the **cochlea duct**.

3. The pressure waves in the endolymph cause the **basilar membrane** to begin to vibrate.

4. This results in the **sensory hair cells** becoming stretched and causes them to produce nerve impulses which are then conducted through the **auditory nerve**.

5. The vibrations of the basilar membrane are conducted

through to the tympanic canal and result in the **round window** vibrating in the air filled middle ear (this allows the vibrations to pass harmlessly out of the cochlea)

(c) The excess mucus produced when a person has a heavy cold can block the **eustachian (auditory) tube** and lead to partial deafness. The eustachian tube allows pressure on each side of the ear drum to be equal. If it is blocked, the air pressure outside the ear and in the middle ear may not be equal, causing the **tympanic membrane** (ear drum) to become taut and unable to vibrate freely.

(d) An **ampulla** is a small swelling found at the base of each semicircular canal. They detect movements of the head and are involved with keeping balance. They are similar to the organ of Corti because they consist of a group of sensory hair cells which give off nerve impulses when they are stretched. In addition to this, the ampulla also contains the fluid endolymph.

Key Words

Neurone (sensory, motor, connector)
Myelin Sheath
Ganglion
Synapse
Nerve Impulse
Reflex
Grey and White Matter
Cerebellum
Cerebral Cortex
Medulla Oblongata
Hypothalamus
Pituitary Gland
Sclera
Choroid
Retina
Rods and Cones
Accommodation
Myopia (short sight)
Hypermetropia (long sight)
Ossicles
Eustachian tube
Cochlea
Ampulla

ANSWER 25

(a) i) and ii)

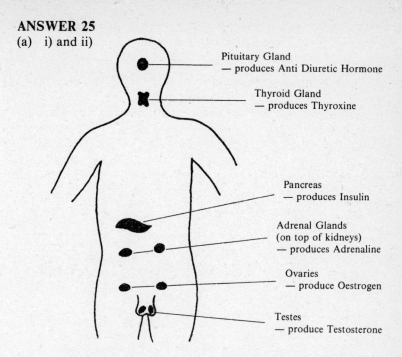

Pituitary Gland
— produces Anti Diuretic Hormone

Thyroid Gland
— produces Thyroxine

Pancreas
— produces Insulin

Adrenal Glands
(on top of kidneys)
— produces Adrenaline

Ovaries
— produce Oestrogen

Testes
— produce Testosterone

The diagram above shows the position in the body of the main endocrine glands along with an example of a hormone produced by the gland.

iii) Hormones all share the following characteristics:—
1. They are chemicals produced by an endocrine gland.
2. They are transported in the blood stream.
3. They act on a particular target organ (or organs), e.g. Anti-Diuretic Hormone only acts on the kidney.

(b) i) In patients suffering from diabetes their pancreas does not produce or cannot release sufficient **insulin**.[1]

ii) Insulin helps to control the blood glucose concentration. An increase in the level of glucose in the blood stimulates the release of insulin from the pancreas. The hormone then causes **glucose** to be taken out of the blood stream and be converted to **glycogen** in the liver and muscles. In this way, insulin causes the concentration of glucose in the blood to fall.

(c) **Adrenaline** is released from the adrenal glands, it causes many changes in the body, including increased heart rate and blood pressure. This is part of "the fight or flight reaction".

1. The pancreas has two functions, one as an endocrine gland, producing the hormone insulin. This is carried out by a group of cells called the **Islets of Langerhans.** Its second function is to produce digestive juices which are passed into the duodenum (this is called an **exocrine** secretion as it is not passed into the blood stream).

ANSWER 26

(a)

Number	Part	Function
1.	Urethra	Allows the passage of semen and urine[1] (but **never** at the same time).
2.	Epididymis	This region is where sperm cells are stored.
3.	Testis	This is the site for the formation of **sperm** and the secretion of the hormone **testosterone.**
4.	Scrotum	This sac of skin supports the testis.
5.	Seminal vesicle	This produces seminal fluid which provides nutrients for the sperm.

(b) This tissue is known as **spongey tissue** and it contains many **sinuses,** which can fill with blood. During sexual arousal the **arterioles** which supply this tissue **dilate** allowing large amounts of blood to flow in. This causes the spongey tissue to become hard and the penis to become erect. This then enables the penis to be inserted into the vagina during sexual intercourse.

(c) The reason why the testes are suspended beneath the trunk of the body in the scrotum, is that they function most effectively at around 35°C. If the testes had not descended, but remained in the abdomen they would have been at normal body temperature i.e. 37°C which would be too hot for sperm production to occur. The result would be that the man would be infertile.

(d) **Sperm** is the name given to the male gametes (sex cells)[2] which are produced by the testes. **Semen** is a liquid which contains sperm and the secretions of the seminal vesicles, cowpers gland and the prostate gland. Semen is the fluid mixture which is ejaculated from the penis, and it may contain up to 100 million sperm cells.[3]

1. This is a very important point, semen and urine **never mix** in the urethra. The penis is unable to carry the two together. This explains why a man cannot urinate when the penis is fully erect.

2. See question 1.

3. The semen ejaculated is made up of over 99½% seminal fluid and less than ½% actual sperm cells by volume.

ANSWER 27
(a) and (b)

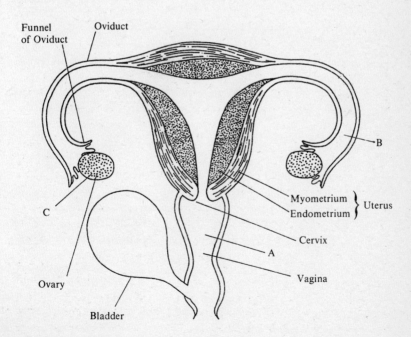

Diagram representing the female reproductive system.

(c)	Oestrogen	Progesterone
	1. Produced by Graafian follicle.	1. Produced by corpus luteum.
	2. Highest blood concentration occurs around the 13th[1] day after menstruation.	2. Highest blood concentration around the 21st[1] day after menstruation.
	3. Its effect is to cause repair and thickening of the endometrium.	3. Its effect is to cause blood vessels to grow into the endometrium (**vascularisation**) and to maintain its thickness.
	4. A fall in the level of oestrogen occurs after ovulation.	4. A fall in the level of progesterone occurs if the ovum has not been fertilised and causes the endometrium to be shed.

(d) Step 1 — **ovulation** can be prevented by the use of the contraceptive pill. This contains a mixture of hormones similar to oestrogen and progesterone which prevent an ovum being released.

Step 2 — Fertilisation can be prevented if the sperm and ovum are kept separate. This could be achieved by the use of a barrier method, such as a diaphragm by the female or a condom (sheath), by the male.

Step 3 — implantation is prevented when the female uses an intra-uterine device (IUD) such as the coil or loop.[2]

1. These figures are often quoted in textbooks, they are simply **average** figures. The **actual** length of the menstrual cycle varies greatly between individuals and also varies in the same individual between different periods.

2. The "morning after" pill (post coital pill) also acts by preventing a fertilised ovum implanting.

ANSWER 28

(a) The sperm would be deposited in the **vagina** before proceeding to swim through the **cervical canal** in the **cervix**. From there it would pass through the **uterus** and into one of the **oviducts (fallopian tubes)**. Fertilisation would take place in the upper third of the oviduct.

(b) i) The term **ovulation** describes the release of a mature ovum from the ovary. This occurs around the 14th day after menstruation commenced. The ovum had been developing inside a **Graafian follicle** until the point of ovulation, where the follicle burst and released the ovum.

  ii) **Fertilisation** is said to have occured when the head of a sperm cell (containing its nucleus) has penetrated the cell membrane of an ovum. The nuclei of the sperm and ovum fuse together to form a **zygote** (fertilised ovum). Fertilisation must normally occur in the uppermost third of the oviduct as an ovum may only be able to survive for between 24-48 hours after ovulation.

  iii) Around a week after fertilisation the zygote has undergone a number of cell divisions and consists of around 20-50 cells. It then digests away a part of the endometrium and becomes embedded. This is known as **implantation**.

(c) i) The **umbilical artery** carries blood from the circulation of the foetus to the **placenta**. The **umbilical vein** carries blood back from the placenta to the foetal circulation.

Umbilical artery	Umbilical vein
1. Low concentration of oxygen.	1. High concentration of oxygen.
2. High concentration of urea.	2. Lower concentration of urea.
3. Low concentration of glucose.	3. Higher concentration of glucose.

  ii) 1. The circulation of the foetus is contained in tiny blood capillaries. If the mother's blood lead directly into these capillaries, her blood pressure would be too high and would cause the capillaries to burst.

2. The mother and foetus may have different blood groups. If their blood mixed freely, this would result in agglutination.

3. The mother's blood contains many hormones which would produce undesirable effects on the development of the foetus, e.g. if it were a male foetus and the blood did mix, the mother's sex hormones would directly affect the foetus.[1]

iii) The foetus has the following adaptations:—

a) Blood flows through the umbilical artery to the placenta and back through the umbilical vein.

b) **Foramen ovale** — this is a small hole which allows blood to flow from the right atrium through into the left atrium. This allows blood to by-pass the lungs which are not functioning.[2]

c) The **ductus arteriosus** is a blood vessel which connects the pulmonary artery to the aorta. Again this allows blood to by-pass the lungs.

Shortly after birth, the vessels in the umbilical constrict (close up), allowing it to be cut with no blood loss. Within a few hours of birth the ductus arteriosus closes and within a few days the foramen ovale also closes.

1. Some other harmful substances present in the mother's blood are capable of passing through the placenta, e.g. Rubella (German Measles) virus, drugs (e.g. thalidomide), or carbon monoxide (from smoking), and alcohol.

2. The lungs are full of **amniotic fluid** and the foetus obtains its oxygen from the placenta.

ANSWER 29

(a) i) A represents fatty (adipose) tissue.

B represents the nipple.

C represents **milk (lactiferous) duct** where milk is stored for a short time.

D represents the **milk lobule** where milk is produced.

ii) **Colostrum** is the thin straw-coloured liquid produced by the mammary glands for the first three or four days after birth.

It is rich in proteins and contains antibodies which may help to prevent the child from contracting gut infections.

iii) Three advantages to the child of breast feeding are:—
1. The milk is sterile and colostrum contains antibodies which may help to prevent gastric infections.
2. The milk is at correct temperature.
3. The milk contains the correct quantities of all nutrients (except iron) needed for a balanced diet.

iv) Human milk contains **no iron,** however a new born baby has large stores of iron which may last for several months.

(b) Both hormones are produced by the pituitary gland, **prolactin** is formed by the anterior lobe and **oxytocin** by the posterior lobe.
Prolactin and oxytocin are involved in the production of milk and its ejection from the mammary glands. **Prolactin** is only produced after birth and causes the **production** of milk to begin. **Oxytocin** is released in a reflex action when the nipple is stimulated and causes milk to be **ejected** from the breast.[1]
Oxytocin is also produced during the latter stages of pregnancy and is involved in the birth process. Oxytocin causes the contraction of the myometrium during labour and birth itself.

(c) i) **Amniocentesis** is a procedure which may be carried out on pregnant women. It involves the removal of a small amount of **amniotic fluid.** This procedure allows the cells of the foetus to be screened for signs of Down's syndrome and spina bifida.

ii) Amniotic fluid supports the foetus and protects it from damage by acting as a shock absorber. It also allows the foetus freedom of movement.

iii) For the first few days the baby receives colostrum which is not as nutritious as milk. Thus the baby uses up some of its stored food supplies and loses weight.

---

1. Milk is not actually sucked from the breast by the action of the baby's mouth. It is ejected by tiny muscles in the walls of the milk ducts and sinuses.

ANSWER 30

(a) i) Between the ages of approximately **9-13 yrs.**

ii) **180cm** is the average height of a fully grown male and **168cm** for a fully grown female.

iii) An average 12 yr. old male would be **132cm.**

iv) The two ages at which males and females are the same average size are around **10 yrs.** and **15½ yrs.** of age. (This corresponds to where the lines for males and females cross over).

(b) i) This stage is known as **puberty.**[2]

ii) The secondary sexual characteristics of the male include:
1. Increase in the size of testes and penis.
2. Testes produce the hormone testosterone[3] and begin the production of sperm.
3. Hair grows on face, underarms, pubic region and generally all over the body.
4. There is a general increase in size of the skeleton and muscles.
5. Psychological changes, i.e. an interest in own appearance plus interest in the opposite sex.
6. The voice deepens due to growth of larynx.

All of these changes are under the control of the hormone testosterone.

(c) The following factors all affect growth:—
1. **Genetics** — i.e. a person inherits genes from their parents which will determine the maximum possible height.
2. **Hormones** — the rate of growth and final height are carefully controlled by hormones, particularly growth hormone (from anterior lobe of pituitary gland).
3. **Diet** — correct amounts of calcium, phosphate and vitamin D are needed for bones to grow correctly.

Exercise can also have some effect on growth. During exercise blood flow to muscles increases. As the muscles are attached to bones, these also receive an increased blood flow which can help to stimulate growth.

---

1. This represents the "flattest" part of the graph where the line is not going up sharply.

2. This should not be confused with adolescence which is not a biological term but refers to a more general phase of emotional changes. Puberty is a biological term and refers specifically to physical and hormonal changes.

3. The testes start producing testosterone after they have been affected by follicle stimulating hormone. The release of FSH from the pituitary gland is the very first stage in puberty.

Key Words
Endocrine
Exocrine
Hormone
Testes
Semen
Sperm
Menstruation
Ovulation
Endometrium
Vascularisation
Graafian follicle
Ovum
Corpus luteum
Fertilisation
Zygote
Implantation
Umbilical cord
Placenta
Amnion
Foramen ovale
Ductus Arteriosus
Amniocentesis
Lactation
Colostrum

ANSWER 31

(a) i) All cells in the body, except erythrocytes and gametes (sex cells) contain 46 chromosomes in their nucleus. Of these, two are known as the sex chromosomes, the remaining 44 (known as autosomes) are made up of 22 pairs of **homologous chromosomes.** A pair of homologous chromosomes consist of two chromosomes of identical shape and length, which carry genes for the same characteristics.

ii) Normally a chromosome consists of a long single strand of **DNA** and **protein.** However shortly before a cell divides, each chromosome shortens and thickens and then makes an identical copy of itself. Thus before cell division, a chromosome consists of two strands called **chromatids** which are joined at a point called the **centromere.**

Centromere ————————————————————< Chromatids

A chromosome before cell division.

iii) During **meiosis** homologous chromosomes line up opposite each other at the spindle. At certain points the chromatids of these homologous chromosomes cross over. The points where this occurs are known as **chiasmata**. At the chiasmata, pieces of chromosomes may be exchanged.[1]

(b) i) There are two major differences between cells produced by **mitosis** and **meiosis:**

      1. Those produced by mitosis contain 46 chromosomes and are said to be **diploid,** whereas those from meiosis contain only 23 chromosomes and are known as **haploid.**[2]

      2. The cells produced by **mitosis** are all **identical** to the parent cell and to each other. Those produced by **meiosis** however all contain **different** combinations of chromosomes to the parent cell and each other.

      Thus meiosis produces **variation** in the daughter cells which contain the haploid number of chromosomes whereas mitosis produces daughter cells with an identical number and combination of chromosomes.

  ii) Meiosis only occurs in the gamete forming organs, i.e. the **testes** and **ovaries.** Mitosis occurs in the majority of body tissues such as the skin or hair.

(c) The sex of an individual is determined by the type of sex chromosomes contained in the cell nuclei. If **two X** chromosomes are present, the person is **female,** if an **X and a Y** chromosome are present, this produces a **male.**

All gametes contain the **haploid** number of chromosomes (i.e. 23) and therefore only contain one sex chromosome. The female ova all contain one X chromosome. Some of the sperm contain an X and others a Y chromosome. Thus the sex of an individual is determined by the type of sperm cell which fertilises the ovum. As there are approximately an equal number of X chromosome and Y chromosome containing sperm, there is an equal chance of a child being female or male.

1. The formation of chiasmata ensures that no two sperm or ova contain identical genes. Thus brothers or sisters are never identical, although they are produced from sperm and ova from the same parents.

2. Gametes contain the haploid number of chromosomes (23) so that when they fuse together, the zygote contains the diploid number (46).

ANSWER 32

(a) i) In this example the **phenotype** of an individual refers to their Rhesus blood group. Thus there are two phenotypes,[1] Rhesus positive blood or Rhesus negative blood. The **genotype**[1] describes the **alleles** which are present to produce the phenotype. If R represents the **(dominant)** allele for Rhesus positive blood group and r represents the **(recessive)** allele for Rhesus negative blood group, the possible genotypes are RR, Rr or rr.

ii) [2]Let R represent the allele for Rhesus positive and r represent the allele for Rhesus negative blood groups.

Parents	Phenotype	Genotype
Mother	Rhesus positive	RR or Rr
Father	Rhesus positive	RR or Rr

The genotype of a person who is Rhesus negative must be rr as this is a recessive condition. Thus the child must be rr, to produce a child of this genotype from two Rhesus positive parents, they must both have Rr genotypes.

Parents genotypes = Rr v Rr

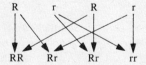

Gametes   R   r   R   r

Possible
Combinations   RR   Rr   Rr   rr

Possible offspring

Genotype: 25% Homozygous dominant (RR)

50% Heterozygous (Rr)

25% Homozygous recessive (rr)

Phenotype: 75% Rhesus positive

25% Rhesus negative

N.B. A simpler, less confusing method of showing possible combinations is to use a table:—

Gametes	R	r
R	RR	Rr
r	Rr	rr

Thus if both parents have Rr genotype they can produce a child who is Rhesus negative. The probability of the child being Rhesus negative is 1 in 4 (25%).

iii)

	Phenotype	Genotype
Mother	Rhesus negative	rr
Baby	Rhesus positive	Rr or RR

For a Rhesus negative mother to produce a Rhesus positive child, the child's father must be Rhesus positive. The father's genotype could be either RR or Rr. As an example the Rr genotype will be used.

Parents genotype = Rr   v   rr

Gametes   Ⓡ ⓡ   ⓡ ⓡ

Possible combinations

Gametes	R	r
r	Rr	rr
r	Rr	rr

Possible offspring
Genotype: 50% Heterozygous (Rr)
                  50% Homozygous recessive (rr)
Phenotype: 50% Rhesus positive
                  50% Rhesus negative

Thus it is possible for a Rhesus negative mother to give birth to a Rhesus positive baby.

iv) A person who is Rhesus negative does not have the Rhesus antigen[3] on their red blood cells. In addition they do not possess any naturally occuring antibodies against the Rhesus antigen in their blood plasma. However, if a Rhesus negative person comes in contact with Rhesus positive blood, they immediately begin producing **anti-Rhesus antibodies.**[4]

During pregnancy or birth, some blood from the foetus leaks into the mother's circulation. If the **baby** is **Rhesus positive** and the **mother** is **Rhesus negative,** this causes the mother to begin producing anti Rhesus antibodies.

These antibodies remain in the mother's bloodstream. If any further children are conceived that are Rhesus positive, the anti-Rhesus antibodies will cross the placenta and cause agglutination of the foetal blood. This results in the foetus becoming anaemic.

1. The Phenotype is the outward appearance of the individual, e.g. blood group, hair colour. The Genotype describes the genes it contains.

2. This question shows a general layout you should use for answering any genetics question. Start by **stating** the information you can obtain from the question, this often helps to clarify things. Then write down the **parents' genotypes** before progressing to the **gametes** and then the **possible combinations**. Finally you should summarise the results of the **offspring** and then answer the question asked, e.g. yes, it is possible for Rhesus positive parents to have Rhesus negative children.

3. See questions 17 and 18.

4. Anti Rhesus antibodies are sometimes known as Anti D.

ANSWER 33

(a) i)   **Incomplete dominance (co-dominance)** occurs where **alleles** are not completely dominant over each other. In the case of blood groups, the alleles for **A** and **B** blood groups are dominant over the allele for **O**. Thus genotypes of **Ao** and **Bo** would produce group A and group B blood respectively. (Where **A** = allele for group A blood, **B** = allele for group B and o = allele for group O). However, when the genotype **AB** occurs, the person does not have type **A** or type **B** blood group but another group called **AB** blood. **AB** blood has has some characteristics of group **A** blood and some of group **B** and is produced by incomplete dominance (co-dominance) between the alleles for **A** and **B** blood groups.

ii) Let A = allele for group A blood.
B = allele for group B blood.
o = allele for group O blood.

Individual	Phenotype (ie blood group)	Genotype
Mother	A	AA or Ao
Child	O	OO
Potential Father	B	BB or Bo

For the mother to give birth to a child of group O, her **genotype** must be **Ao**. If the father who is blood group B has the **genotype Bo**, the child could be his. This can be shown by the possible offspring from this couple given below:—

Parents' genotypes = Ao   v   Bo.
Gametes =   Ⓐ ⓞ   Ⓑ ⓞ

Gametes	B	o
A	AB	Ao
o	Bo	oo

Possible offspring
Genotypes: 25% Heterozygous AB
                25% Heterozygous Ao
                25% Heterozygous Bo
                25% Homozygous oo
Phenotypes: 25% Blood group AB
                25% Blood group A
                25% Blood group B
                25% Blood group O

Thus it can be seen that this man of group B blood **could be** the father of the child with blood group O.

(b) i) The genes for certain conditions such as **haemophilia** and **red-green colour blindness** are carried on the **X-chromosome**. Any gene which occurs on a sex chromosome is said to be a **sex-linked gene.**[1]

   ii) A man not suffering from haemophilia must have the allele for normal clotting H on his X chromosome and would have a genotype X^HY. There are two possible genotypes for a female who does not have haemophilia, X^HX^H where she has two alleles for normal clotting. Alternatively a female could have one allele for normal clotting and one for haemophilia, that is an X^HX^h genotype.

   iii) Because haemophilia is a **recessive** condition, some women may have normal blood clotting and also contain the allele for haemophilia. These women would have an X^HX^h **genotype** and are said to be carriers.

Let X^H = allele for normal clotting
X^h = allele for haemophilia

Parents	Phenotype	Genotype
Father	Normal clotting	$X^H Y$
Mother	Carrier female	$X^H X^h$

Parents genotype = $X^H Y$ v $X^H X^h$

Gametes = X^H Y X^H X^h

Possible combinations

Gametes	X^H		Y	
X^H	X^H	X^H	X^H	Y
X^h	X^H	X^h	X^h	Y

Possible offspring

Genotypes: 25% $X^H X^H$
25% $X^H X^h$
25% $X^H Y$
25% $X^h Y$

Phenotypes: 25% Normal female
25% Carrier female
25% Normal male
25% Haemophiliac male

Thus if a carrier female and a normal male have children, they could produce offspring with the possible phenotypes shown above.

1. Sex linked genes are very rarely carried on the Y chromosome. Virtually all those sex linked characteristics which you will encounter will be associated with the X chromosome.

Key Words	
Deoxyribonucleic Acid (DNA)	Gene
Chromosome	Allele
Homologous pair	Dominant
Chromatid	Recessive
Centromere	Homozygous
Sex chromosome	Heterozygous
Mitosis	Carrier
Meiosis	Sex linked
Chiasmata	Incomplete dominance
Diploid	Rhesus positive
Haploid	Rhesus negative
Genotype	Haemophilia
Phenotype	Red-Green colour blindness

ANSWER 34

(a) **Sewage** consists of human urine and faeces whereas **refuse** is made up of all the items and materials that man throws away, e.g. potato peelings, bones etc.

(b) **Refuse** is buried for the following reasons:—
1. This prevents pests such as rodents, birds and houseflies from feeding off it.
2. Saprophytic[1] micro-organisms in the soil decompose much of the organic waste.
3. During decomposition, unpleasant odours may be released, these can be minimised by burying the refuse.
4. Organic waste may be a source of **pathogens,**[2] burying the waste reduces the chances of these being passed on to man by vectors such as rodents etc.

(c) i) The soil contains saprophytic micro-organisms which break down the organic waste.

ii) The remaining 40% is likely to consist of materials which can not be decomposed by micro-organisms in the soil, e.g. plastics, bottles, etc.

(d) There are a number of different forms of sewage treatment, but they all follow basically the same sequence of events. The main stages are described below:—
1. **Screening**
As the liquid enters the treatment process, it is passed through a series of wire meshes. These remove solid objects such as babies' nappies, cans etc.
2. **Grit settlement**
The liquid is allowed to flow very slowly along narrow channels. This allows heavy particles such as grit to settle out. The grit is periodically removed, washed and then used for purposes such as road building.
3. **Sedimentation Tanks**
The sewage passes into large sedimentation (or settlement) tanks where it is allowed to stand for up to 10 hours. In this time, suspended solids settle at the bottom of the tank[3] to form settled (or primary) **sludge.** The sludge is rapidly removed and passed into sludge digestion tanks.

4. **Sludge Digester**

    This consists of large tanks containing sludge. The tanks are not aerated which encourages the growth of **anaerobic bacteria** which digest the sludge and release **methane gas.** The gas is collected and can be sold or used to power the pumps in the sewage works. The digested sludge can then be dried out and sold as fertiliser.

5. **Aeration tanks**[4]

    The liquid effluent from the sedimentation tanks is passed into large ponds. In these tanks air is bubbled through the liquid which is constantly stirred. This encourages the growth of **aerobic bacteria** which digest organic waste and causes the build up of sponge-like network of **activated sludge.** The activated sludge also contains **protozoa** (single called animals) and **fungi** which help to break down any pathogenic micro-organism still in the effluent.

6. **Biological Filter**[5]

    These consist of beds of coke and stones. The effluent is spread over the coke beds by a rotating sprinkler. The coke and stones are covered by a **film of micro-organisms** including **protozoa** and aerobic bacteria which digest any organic debris or pathogens in the effluent.

7. **Humus Tanks**

    Finally before the **effluent** is released into rivers and lakes, it is allowed to stand in large **humus** tanks. Here any small particles, or organic debris from the biological filter, settles out. The humus is regularly removed and may provide a source of activated sludge, or may be dried and used as a fertiliser.

1. Saprophytic micro-organisms feed off dead or decaying organic material.

2. A pathogen is a micro-organism that causes a disease in man. (NB. The word **Germs** should <u>never</u> be used in biology. If used in an exam you will be penalised).

3. In some cases, sedimentation is accelerated by the addition of a chemical (ferric chloride) which causes flocculation (i.e. small particles to stick together).

4. Sewage works using this technique are said to be using the activated sludge method.

5. Most older sewage works used only this technique rather than the activated sludge method.

ANSWER 35

(a) **Potable water** is drinking water which is free from chemicals and pathogens. It should not contain, soil particles, industrial wastes, undesirable tastes or odours.

(b) i) During the purification of water, sedimentation allows large particles to settle out. Water is held in large storage tanks to allow this process to occur. Chemicals may be added to speed up sedimentation. The chemicals cause small particles to stick together (flocculate).

    ii) The slow sand filter consists of layers of fine sand, coarse sand and gravel. The upper layer of the filter is covered by a **jelly or slime layer** which contains **algae** and **saprophytic bacteria.** The micro-organisms in this slime layer breaks down organic material and pathogens which may be present in the water.

    iii) Any pathogens remaining after filtration can be killed by the addition of **chlorine** to the water. When dissolved in water, chlorine forms a compound (hypochlorous acid) which is highly toxic to micro-organisms.

(c) i) **Cholera** and **typhoid** fever can both be spread by contaminated water.

    ii) If large amounts of untreated sewage were added to a river, it would be decomposed by bacteria. The bacteria involved are **aerobic** and therefore they use up oxygen dissolved in the water whilst decomposing the organic material. This results in the level of **dissolved oxygen** in the river **falling.** Eventually the level of oxygen remaining will not be sufficient for the animal life in the river to survive.

(d) i) If food scraps are not wrapped before being placed in a dustbin, they give off an unpleasant odour as they decompose. This may attract pests, such as rodents, or flies to the bin. In addition to this, any organic material provides a site where houseflies can lay their eggs. Thus it is important to wrap up food scraps to prevent pests gaining access.

    ii) All raw meat, including a chicken, contains some bacteria. If a chicken is cooked from frozen, although the outside may be well done, the inside will not cook thoroughly. Thus the inside of the chicken will be **warm** and **moist,** ideal conditions for **bacterial growth.** The increased number of bacteria could then produce food poisoning in a person eating the chicken.

ANSWER 36

(a) i) The addition of salt to preserve food is an example of **osmotic preservation.** As the salt soaks into the food it raises its osmotic pressure. Any micro-organisms which then land on the salted food become dehydrated as water is drawn out of them by **osmosis.**

ii) Before food is canned it is cooked to destroy micro-organisms that could cause decay. Then, while still hot, it is placed into cans and the lid is sealed. The cans are then rapidly cooled, causing the contents to shrink and producing a **partial vacuum** in the can. Once sealed, the can is airtight and therefore micro-organisms cannot enter.

iii) During pickling, vinegar (which is mainly acetic acid), is added to foods. This stops food from spoiling as the acid prevents the growth of bacteria.

(b) The essential difference between high temperature treatment and refrigeration is that, bacteria are **killed** by **high temperatures** but simply made **inactive** by refrigeration. Thus, if food is cooked thoroughly first, most bacteria that might cause food spoilage are killed and the food will last for some time. If the same food had not been cooked but placed in a refrigerator instead, it would not have been preserved as long. During refrigeration the bacterial spoilage of the food would simply be slowed down, not stopped.

(c) **Freezing does not kill** bacteria, it simply renders them inactive. Bacteria can grow and reproduce rapidly between a temperature range of between $10°C - 65°C$. A freezer produces temperatures between $- 6°C$ to $- 24°C$. A freezer produces reduce bacterial action. As food is de-frosted, the temperature rises gradually and bacteria begin to reproduce. Food, particularly meat, should be eaten as soon after defrosting as possible. If this food were re-frozen, then the increased number of bacteria will again become inactive. When this food is defrosted for the second time, the bacteria again reproduce very rapidly. The result of this is that after the second defrosting the number of bacteria in the food may be sufficiently high to produce food poisoning in any person consuming it.

(d) The following procedures could help to control the spread of diseases by houseflies.
  1. All food scraps should be wrapped before being thrown away. This removes a possible food supply and site for egg laying from the fly.
  2. All food should be kept covered or left in a refrigerator to prevent houseflies landing and contaminating it.
  3. All dustbins should have tight-fitting lids and should be disinfected regularly.
  4. Insecticidal sprays can be used to kill adult flies but should be used with caution, as they may be harmful to man or animals.

ANSWER 37

(a) i) Cereal crop ⟶ slug ⟶ Thrush ⟶ Hawk.

  ii) An example of a **producer** is the cereal crop. This crop is eaten by a mouse which is therefore a **primary consumer (herbivore).** The mouse in turn may be eaten by a hawk which is therefore a **secondary consumer (carnivore).**

  iii) The ultimate source of energy for this and all food webs is **sunlight.**

(b) The energy from sunlight is made available to man in the following stages:—
  1. Initially the sunlight energy is used by the cereal crop to carry out **photosynthesis.** During this process a simple food molecule such as **glucose** is produced.

$$6\,CO_2 \;+\; 6\,H_2O \xrightarrow{\text{sunlight + chlorophyll}} C_6H_{12}O_6 \;+\; 6\,O_2$$

| $6\,CO_2$ | $6\,H_2O$ | $C_6H_{12}O_6$ | $6\,O_2$ |
| Carbon Dioxide | Water | Glucose | Oxygen |

[1]

The glucose formed is then stored by the plant as a more complex molecule such as **starch.**

2. Man then consumes the cereal, and it is **digested** in the alimentary canal. The starch is broken down into glucose which is then absorbed into the bloodstream.

3. The glucose is taken up by the cells and broken down during **respiration** to release energy. Thus the sun's energy originally used to synthesise glucose in the plant, is then released during respiration in a human cell.

(c) The level of oxygen in the air surrounding the cereal crop will be affected by two processes which occur in plant cells, **photosynthesis** and **respiration.** During respiration, oxygen is removed from the air and used for the breakdown of glucose to release energy.

$$C_6H_{12}O_6 + 6 O_2 \longrightarrow 6 CO_2 + 6 H_2O + Energy$$
Glucose + Oxygen $\qquad\qquad$ Carbon Dioxide + water + energy

Respiration will take place in all the plant cells throughout the day.

During the hours of daylight **photosynthesis** takes place. In this process carbon dioxide is removed from the air and oxygen is released.

$$6CO_2 + 6H_2O \xrightarrow{\text{chlorophyll} + \text{sunlight}} C_6H_{12}O_6 + 6O_2$$
Carbon + Water $\qquad\qquad$ Glucose + Oxygen
Dioxide

Thus in daylight, photosynthesis occurs at a much faster rate than respiration. The result is that oxygen will be released into the air.

At **night,** although the plant cells will **still** be **respiring,** they will have stopped carrying out photosynthesis. The net result will be that oxygen is removed from the air.

Thus in summary, the oxygen concentration in the air is likely to be **highest** during daylight and **lowest** at night.

(d) i) Nitrogen is an essential [2]component of **amino acids.** All organisms contain proteins and therefore they all contain the element nitrogen.

ii) The following are the bacteria involved with the nitrogen cycle:—

    1. **Nitrogen fixing bacteria** — these are found in the root nodules of leguminous plants. They remove nitrogen from the air and convert it to simple organic molecules (e.g. amino acids).

    2. **Denitrifying bacteria** — These break down nitrates in the soil to release free nitrogen into the atmosphere.

    3. **Nitrifying bacteria** — These convert ammonia into nitrates in the soil. Ammonia is released when dead organic remains decompose.

1. Some O level syllabi in human biology do not require the knowledge of chemical symbols. However, it is very useful to learn the two chemical equations used in this question, i.e. respiration and photosynthesis.

2. This question also explains why plants are removed from a hospital ward at night. In the day they release oxygen into the ward but at night they remove oxygen from the air and release carbon dioxide.

Key Words

Pathogen	Refuse
Aerobic Bacteria	Sewage
Anaerobic Bacteria	Screening
Nitrogen Fixing Bacteria	Settlement
Denitrifying Bacteria	Sedimentation
Nitrifying Bacteria	Sludge
Saprophyte	Aeration tank
Protozoa	Biological Filter
Fungi	Humus
Producer	Effluent
Primary consumer (herbivore)	Potable water
Secondary consumer (carnivore)	Dissolved oxygen
Photosynthesis	Chlorine
Respiration	Humus